TIEVE TARA

BY

Dr. Richard Sloan

Grosvenor House
Publishing Limited

This book is published by
Grosvenor House Publishing Ltd
Link House
140 The Broadway, Tolworth, Surrey, KT6 7HT.
www.grosvenorhousepublishing.co.uk

A CIP record for this book
is available from the British Library

ISBN 978-1-83975-220-9

This book is dedicated to my late wife

Kathleen Mary Sloan

1946–2015

Tieve Tara Medical Centre Practice Manager

About the author

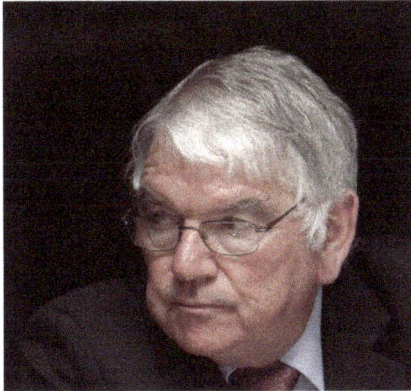

Richard Sloan has at least twenty-two doctors in his family. He was born in Leeds and brought up in Tieve Tara, Airedale, Castleford, attending school first in Airedale and then Queen Elizabeth Grammar School, Wakefield. He was a medical student first at University College London, and then The London Hospital Medical College. After qualifying as a doctor, he obtained a PhD for three years' work on human temperature regulation as a lecturer in Physiology. He became a general practitioner in Cheltenham, Gloucestershire, and then at Tieve Tara, Airedale, Castleford. He was nominated FRCGP in 2002 and awarded an MBE for Services to Medicine and Healthcare in West Yorkshire in 2011. He is a trustee of three charities: Healthwatch Wakefield, Spectrum People and Age UK Wakefield.

Contents

Acknowledgements

I have two people to thank for my writing this book.

The first is my friend, Steve Shalet. Steve was a medical student with me at The London Hospital Medical College. He is an eminent endocrinologist and Emeritus Professor of Endocrinology at the Christie Hospital at Manchester. We have kept in touch for more than fifty years. In 2017 I visited him in Derbyshire, and he showed me a three-page essay he had written about his daughter. He suggested I wrote one about my mother. When we next met at my house, I showed him my essay and he gave me some very positive feedback. The discipline of having to stick to three pages makes one self-edit, prioritise and only allow limited rambling on. (I am an expert at the latter as you will see.) It was writing two or three of these essays that got me thinking about this book.

I was contacted by the National Association of Primary Care (NAPC) in June 2018 to write something about my memories of the NHS as a child and teenager living with my parents in the 1950s and also thoughts about the NHS for which I worked for over forty years. The second person I want to thank is Ann Knight, communications consultant of the NAPC. She edited my contribution and was motivating and positive about my memories and thoughts. It was because of that I decided to write this book.

Thank you to Grosvenor House publishing for wise advice and for publishing this book.

I am grateful to Hannah Jones, freelance proofreader, for an excellent job. (www.theremedyoferrors.com)

Introduction

The house, Tieve Tara, was so named by my father and his first wife in 1923. It was built by Fryston Colliery especially for my father and his family. He was its colliery doctor. He rented at first and, after a couple of years, bought it. The Sloans were Irish. The meaning of Tieve is house and is derived from Gaelic. A few girls have a Christian name of Tieve. The hill of Tara was the seat of the Kings of Ireland from 5000 BC to the eighth century AD and later. Tara can be translated as Queen. It is a popular girl's Christian name. It had a small surgery and then further extensions over the next eighty or so years. Both the house and surgery were called Tieve Tara and the post for each was delivered in one batch. The surgery was and still is semi-detached from the house. The hugely enlarged surgery was renamed Tieve Tara Medical Centre in 2004 and the house renamed Hill House when I retired in 2005. I am pleased that the name lives on.

But where is the hill? There are two approaches to this property and both involve going up a slight incline. The private house is on Airedale Drive and a road serves it and six other properties. Airedale Drive starts with an incline and ends about 20-plus metres above the main road and the neighbouring Fryston village. The first section of road is concreted. The second section was a rough track with potholes. This was tarmacked in 2018. Before about 1981, the surgery was approached by an unmade track from the council estate and from what was one of the most deprived streets in Castleford – Park Dale.

My family translated Tieve Tara as the House on the Hill.

I am writing this book for the patients who have passed through Tieve Tara Surgery/Medical Centre since the early 1920s. It is also for those who have worked there and those who have been associated with the practice. It is a personal reflection and I apologise if I leave something or someone out. The book is also a celebration for me as on 1 November 1978 (just over forty years ago) Tieve Tara Surgery was started up again by me and my wife, Kathleen. My mother had retired in 1976 and the house and surgery were empty and unused.

I find writing therapeutic. All money that is raised from selling this book will go to the charities CAFOD (Catholic Agency for Overseas Development) and Children of Peace. Self-publishing is a marvellous thing, in my opinion, as it gives one freedom. I suspect strongly that not many people will be interested in the photo of my great-grandmother or the detailed description of the new surgery building. However, this is my way of making sure these people and things live on. Some of the public may be interested in how things were in general practice over the years and in learning about the tremendous team effort that is involved. The book gives a view of what goes on behind the scenes in general practice life. It is a history of general practice from a particular viewpoint.

I semi-self-published a book in 2012. It is called "The English Doctor". Some of what I wrote in that book is repeated here from a different angle. This book can be obtained from Amazon in soft or hard copy or downloaded to a Kindle. The royalties from sales have been donated to the charities mentioned above. It is about my medical journey through being a medical student, house officer, research physiologist, GP in Cheltenham, GP trainer, Continuing Medical Education tutor, GP trainee course organiser, associate director of postgraduate GP education, and Primary Care Trust GP education advisor and appraisal lead.

This book is a comment on how a middle-class medical family living in a beautiful house and garden integrated with mainly working-class people attending the surgery next door.

I hope the thoughts, memories and anecdotes in this book capture what general practice was all about for my family living in Tieve Tara house as well as what those buildings meant for patients, friends, staff and others. The NHS might have been reorganised many times since 1948, but Tieve Tara Surgery/Medical Centre will soon have been caring for the patients of Airedale for 100 years.

This book is not just about a building. It is about health inequality; class; teamwork; loyalty; love; friendship; relationships; caring; curing; dying; teaching; joy and laughter; sadness and tears; the future of primary care.

Chapter 1 – The Building

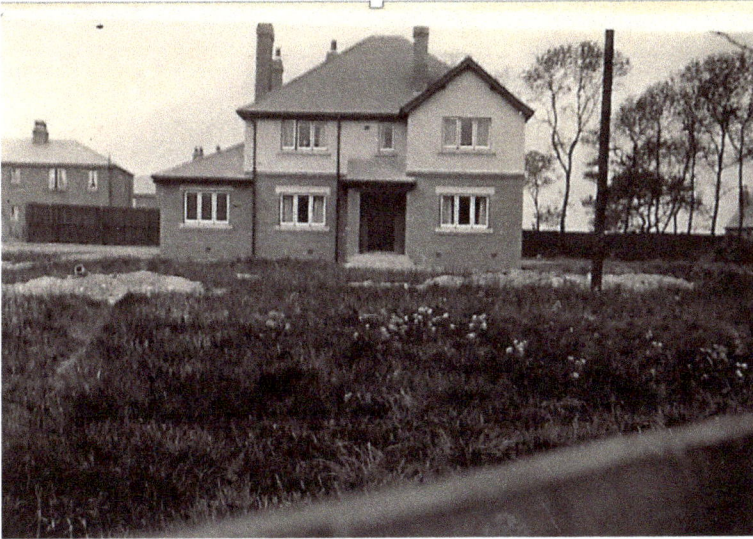

Tieve Tara in 1924

The single-storey extension on the left was a very small surgery. The houses on the left in the background were council houses in Park Dale. Park Dale was a beautiful street in those early years, and my father rented a house there until he could move in to Tieve Tara.

Tieve Tara house had five bedrooms, a bathroom, a kitchen, scullery area, a pantry, dining and sitting rooms and quite an extensive yard and garden. There were electric bell pushes in the dining room and sitting room that could be used to call a maid or housekeeper from the kitchen and scullery. There was no garage for a number of years and my father had to walk to a neighbour's where his car was garaged. This was not a pleasant experience in the middle of the winter at 2 am.

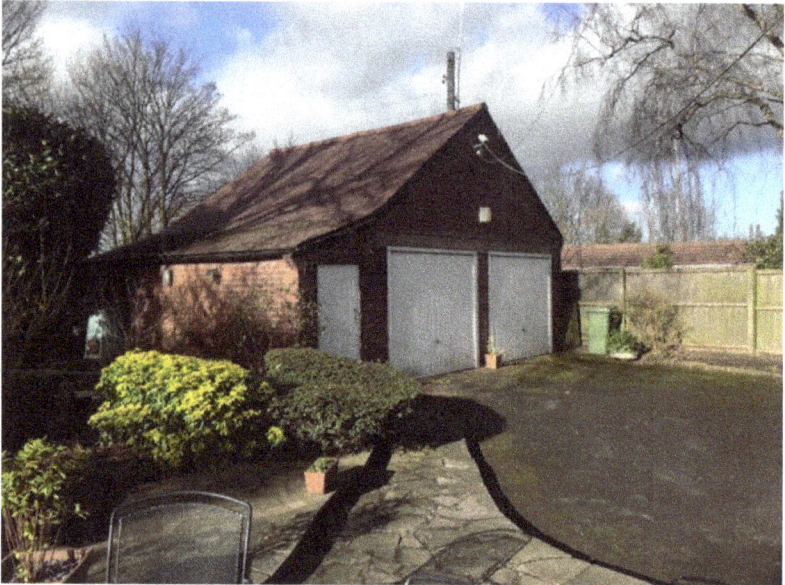

The double garage 2019

I believe the present garage was built by Bill Hirst shortly after my parents' marriage. It is huge. In the 1950s and 1960s there was an electric heater on cold winter nights to prevent the car radiators freezing.

The main garage has two small storage rooms. The door to one can be seen on the left. When I was a lad this was a gang hut for me and my friends. A brick could be removed to create a spyhole to the outside. When I was given a car by my parents in 1963 (a Hillman Imp), there was enough room for me to park it between my parents' cars in the big garage. Soon after that they had a third garage erected for my car. That garage was still there in 1978 when we moved in. My wife, Kath, and I were sometimes a daydreaming team. In the early days we started planning to convert the garage to a restaurant. We even worked out the menus.

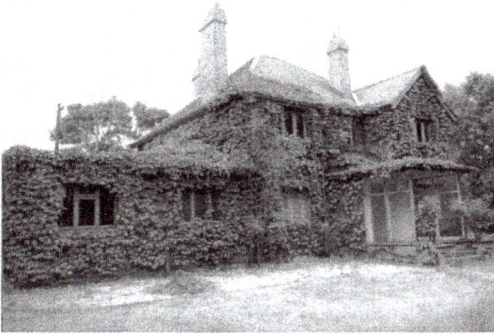

Tieve Tara 1978

This photo was taken the year Kath and I bought the house and surgery from my mother. My mother had the idea of having a veranda built. It was a very European thing in those days. This was a lovely place to be on a warm summer's day. It faced the rose garden and front lawn. I am not sure when the first surgery extension was built. It had two consulting rooms, a waiting room and what was called the dispensary. Well before the NHS (1948), the doctors made up medications and ointments in this room. After the NHS was established, the room was used by the receptionist/typist and contained the patient records. It was also used to test urine etc.

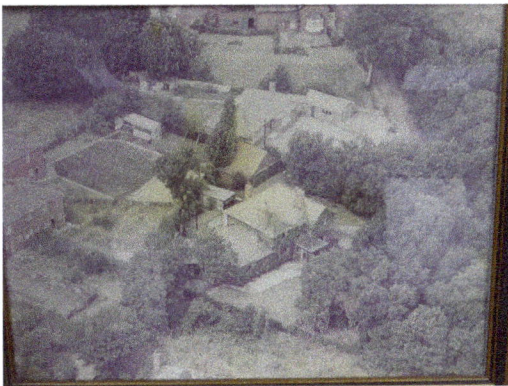

Aerial photo c 1981

This is a framed aerial photograph which we gave to Tieve Tara Surgery many years ago. You may have to use a magnifying glass to follow the next description. The photo shows the house and surgery (semi-detached on the left) just below the centre of the photo, with the veranda in front. The surgery had a flat roof, which was a great place to climb to when I was young. If one laid flat on one's stomach, it was a fantastic hiding place. The last time I climbed up there was when I was about 35 years old.

The surgery was that size from the 1940s to when we had the first extension built in the 1980s.

In 1960 this article was published in the Yorkshire Post:

"ALDERMAN HAD TO WAIT IN RAIN – Doctors asked to review their surgery accommodation.

A Castleford Alderman had to wait in a 60-strong queue outside a Castleford doctor's surgery in the rain for nearly an hour because of extremely inadequate surgery accommodation, it was alleged at the West Riding Health Executive Council at Wakefield yesterday."

At that time, the three partners (my parents and Dr. A. B. C. Smith) had about 10,000 patients.

Soon afterwards, the Pontefract and Castleford Express had the headline:

"EXTRA SURGERY ACCOMMODATION NOT NEEDED AT AIREDALE"

The Executive Council was on the partners' side because it was an isolated occurrence in an influenza epidemic.

Of course it was too small! So it was OK to queue up in the rain with flu!

It is worth pointing out that in 2019 there is a nationwide problem of patients having great difficulty in getting an appointment with a GP. Patients have started arriving at the surgery at

7 am (and in all weathers) to wait outside until the gate and front door are opened a little later on. The queuing outside continues.

The land alongside the left perimeter fence was used to build the first and second surgery extensions. A single garage that was for my car (mentioned above) can be seen to the left of the large double garage, top centre. There is a fence behind those garages extending to join the end of the left perimeter fence. Next door to that fence is a huge garden of a council house rented by Martin and Maud Raftery. Maud's parents, Mr. and Mrs. Bruin, lived there when I was a child and they kept ducks behind that fence. The house to the left of the Raftery's was that of the Wards. Frank Ward was a childhood friend. His brother was called Harold and his mother Muriel. I think his father had a built-up shoe because of a club foot. Muriel used to come out every late afternoon and call "Harold" in a very loud voice to get him to come in for his tea.

A rough road can be seen top right and this is Airedale Drive. In the early 1980s there were six houses, five of which were originally built for senior people working at Fryston Colliery. These were the manager, the bookkeeper, the doctor and two under-managers. Next door to the right of our big garage, a new bungalow was built for Edgar Williams when he retired as a local pit manager.

At the top end of the left perimeter fence there is a large green gate that opens on to the track that leads from Park Dale to the surgery entrance. There was some room to park at the surgery, but the track was full of potholes.

I decided to write round to people to ask for contributions to surface the "back track". Below is one of the letters I received:

16th April 1980

Dear Dr. Sloan,

Thank you for your letter of
22nd February which I got some time
ago, - I was abroad when it arrived
or I would have answered sooner.

I am happy to send you a cheque
for £10 to help you with your project.

Yours sincerely,

Henry Moore

Letter from Henry Moore

The idea of the fund was one of my many crackers ideas and, in the end, we paid to get it surfaced.

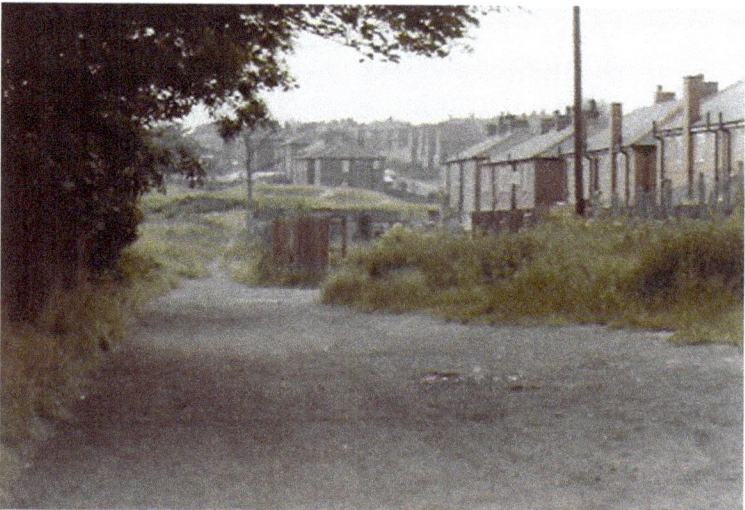

Surgery approach before surfacing (view from surgery)

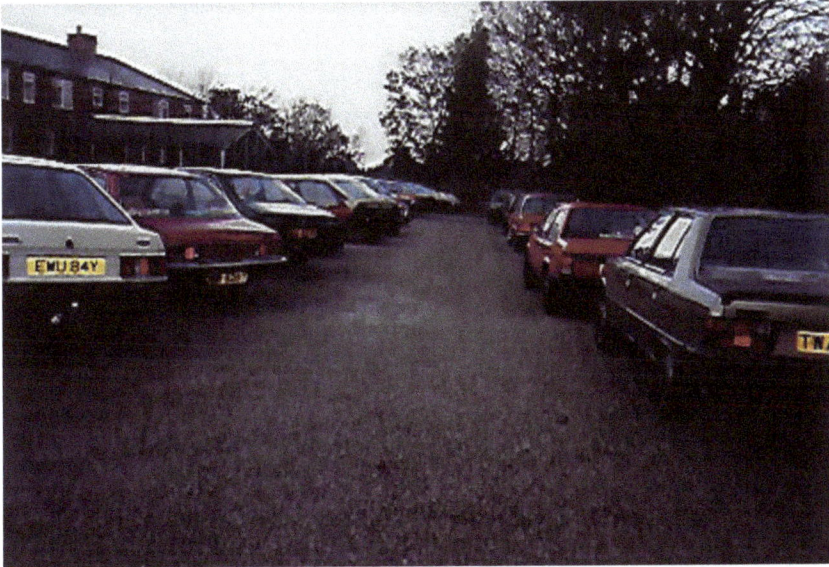

Surgery approach after surfacing (view towards surgery)

In the early 1980s, the then practice manager, my wife, Kathleen, noticed that the cost rent scheme for GP practices for new building projects had new funds which were available. She applied and we had an extension built in our garden. This was the best financial deal imaginable for me and Kath. We had bought the house and surgery from my mother. I and my new partner, John Lee, with a loan from the cost rent scheme, bought the end of our garden for the same amount as we had paid my mother. In effect Kath and I paid no capital for the house and surgery. The cost rent scheme allowed a rent to be calculated that usually was the same as the interest on the cost of the new extension. A few years later we had a second extension and finally in 2004 there was a huge refurbishment and extension towards Park Dale. The latter involved a loan approaching £2 million. I cannot find any photographs of the first two extensions. However, the photograph below from my garden is of the first and second extensions in what was our garden next to the left perimeter fence as mentioned above. The conservatory on the right replaced the veranda.

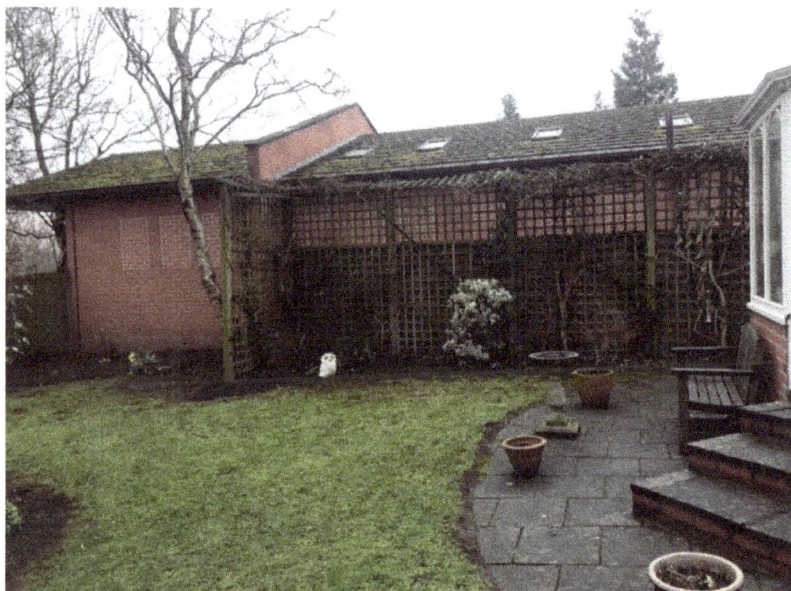

Earlier extensions

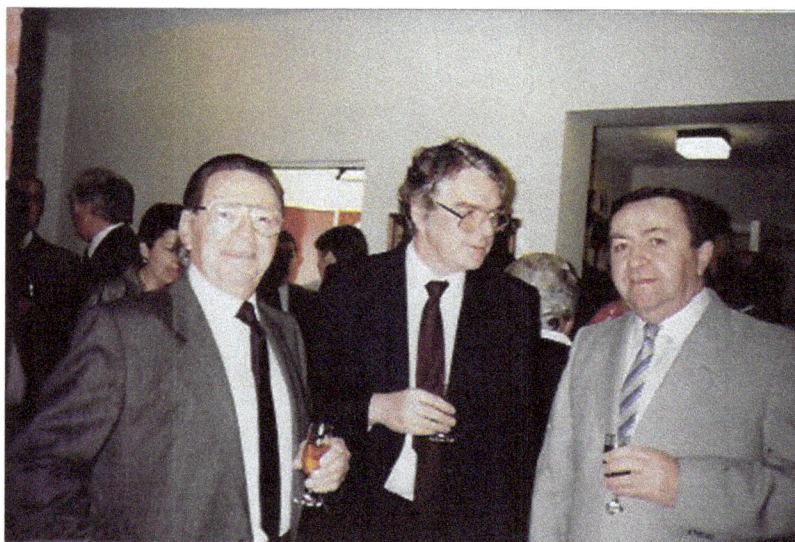

The official opening of the second extension by Sir Jack Smart, Leader, Wakefield Council (left) and Bill Hopwood, Chief Executive, Wakefield Health Authority (right). I am in the middle.

I made a video of the building progress of the huge 2004 extension which is on YouTube. To view, copy this onto a browser: https://youtu.be/3Cgp3fPxDiU It shows the inside of the second extension of the surgery and how cramped we were. It also shows the two portacabins we had before this extension was completed. One was for the practice development manager, Celia, and the other was the practice library and a sitting room. I am sure we were breaking the Factory Act by having staff working in such conditions. I shared my consulting room with our trainee for about a year. I first shared with Sarah Bodey. She was expressing breast milk for her first baby at that time (in private!). Then I shared with Deborah Hewitt.

In the middle of the video I show the opening ceremony for the new College Lane surgery refurbishment and development at Ackworth, Pontefract. Ackworth is about 6 miles away. I had close colleagues there (the main one being Liz Moulton). The Ackworth surgery was built to plans made by the same architect as ours (Spawforths, near Wakefield). It has a beautiful glass entrance and foyer close to the street. That would have lasted a week in Airedale. We had significant vandalism at the start of the building works. A dumper truck was burned out (costing £50,000) and the fencing pulled down (by children). We had to employ an on-site security firm every night for the rest of the work. We had a surrounding high metal fence built. One can see on the video children aged about twelve vandalising the perimeter. One of the neighbours of the practice reported this and someone from Wakefield and District Housing visited the parents and threatened eviction if this behaviour continued. It stopped immediately.

The 2004 building is very large and its size difficult to show using photographs. A patient using the surgery might only see reception, a waiting room and a consulting room and nothing else. I want to show what facilities and rooms there are in a modern GP practice. There is very much more to the 2004 build-ing that patients have never seen. I will now describe Tieve Tara Medical Centre in detail using photographs I have recently taken.

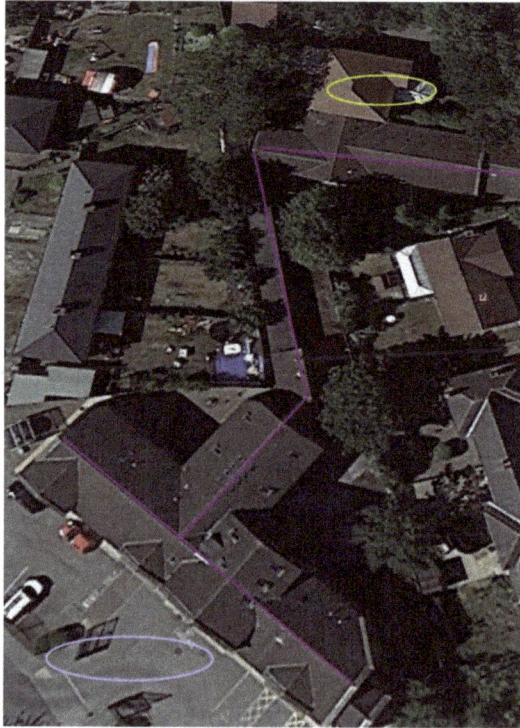

Aerial view February 2019. Thanks to Google Earth for this image.

The yellow ellipse marks Hill House. The blue ellipse is the car park. The purple line shows the extent of the building.

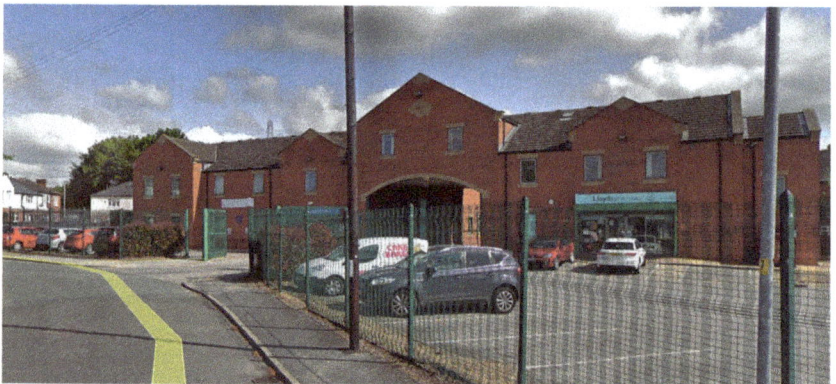

View from Park Dale 2019

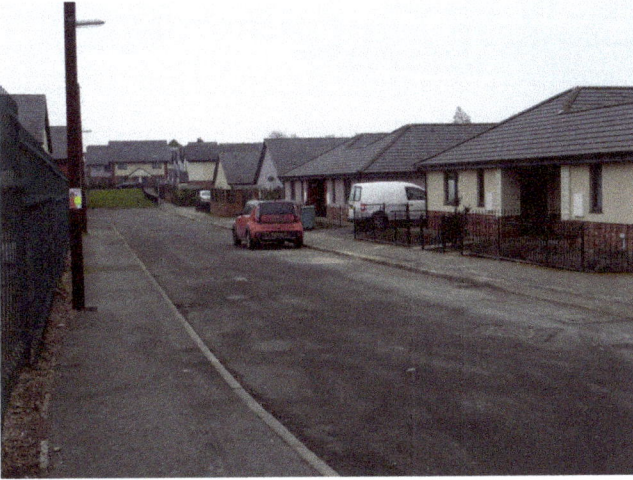

Park Dale 2019 with new eco houses

Most of the Park Dale area was demolished and replaced by modern eco-houses shown above. The council decided to name a street after my family. Kath and I were very proud of this.

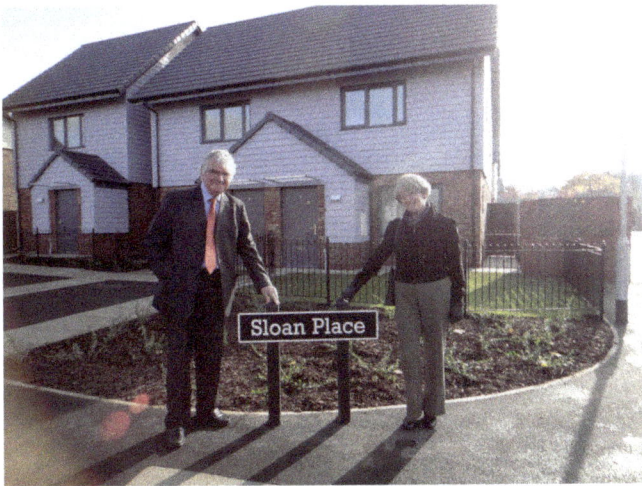

Kath and me at Sloan Place

Kath and I were invited to the official opening of this new development. The main guest was Paul Hudson, a meteorologist who presents the weather forecast for the BBC's Look North. I had to say a few words after him. There were some students present from the Airedale Academy. During my speech one of the girls started to faint and had to be taken outside by a nurse. Paul Hudson told me she fainted because my speech was so boring! I pointed out that faints take time to build up and that it was a reaction to what he said.

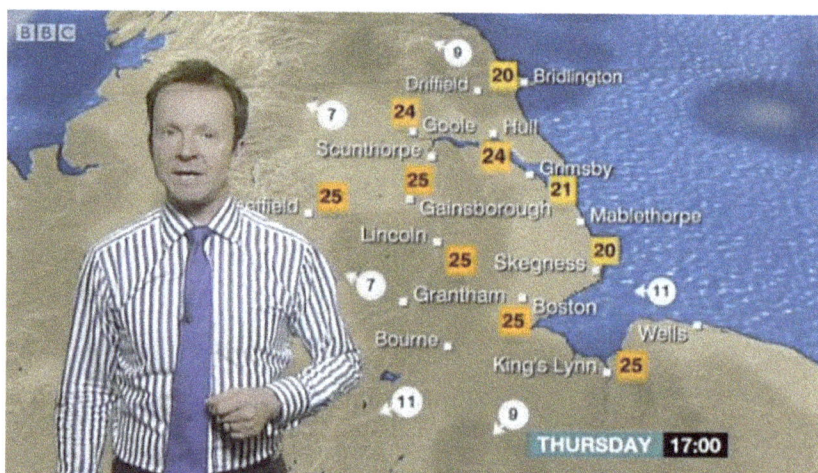

Paul Hudson

At the top of the aerial view, one can see Tieve Tara house with the white-painted conservatory projecting to the right. The red-tiled Tieve Tara house (renamed Hill House after I retired) is semi-detached from the grey tiled refurbished building that was the first extension. This part runs (to the right) close to and parallel to the fence of the next-door bungalow, Oratova, which also has a white framed conservatory projecting from its rear. At the left end of that extension is a long corridor built on the "back track" (the original approach to the surgery). This corridor connects to the main building. The main building has a huge car park. The front of the main building is shown in the view from Park Dale above.

There is an integral chemist, originally Lloyds, which is now owned by another company. The pharmacy pays rent to the surgery. There is also a broad U-shaped opening in the middle of the building. The neighbours behind the clinic always had access to Park Dale and have access now through that connection. They have keys to enable them to get out when the surgery is closed. A look at the video will give you a better picture of this.

One excellent feature of the new build is the large car park. It has capacity for all those visiting the clinic and pharmacy as well as an area for staff-only parking. Meetings of other organisations can be held there.

* * *

I will now take you on a photographic tour of the inside of the surgery/clinic. Walking through the front door of the main entrance, reception is on the left after a corridor that leads to five consulting rooms. Next to reception is the main waiting room.

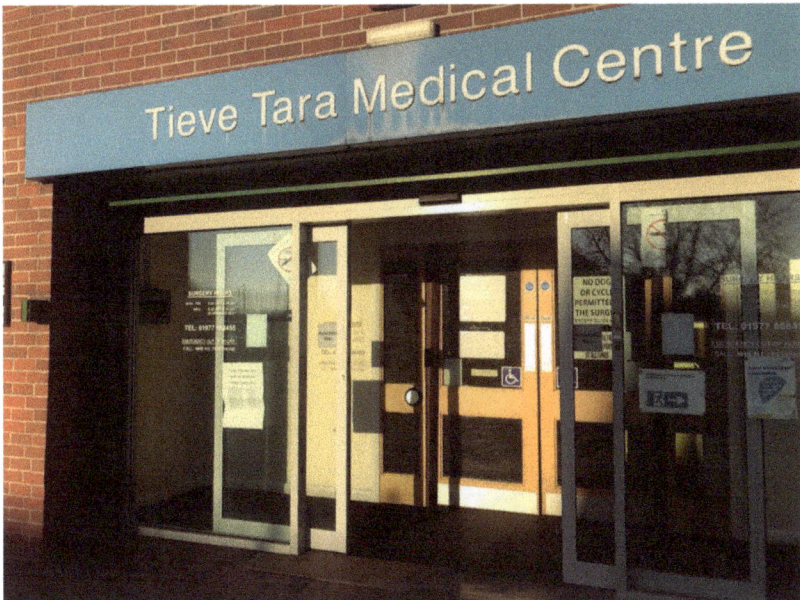

The main entrance

Reception is found immediately after entering the building.

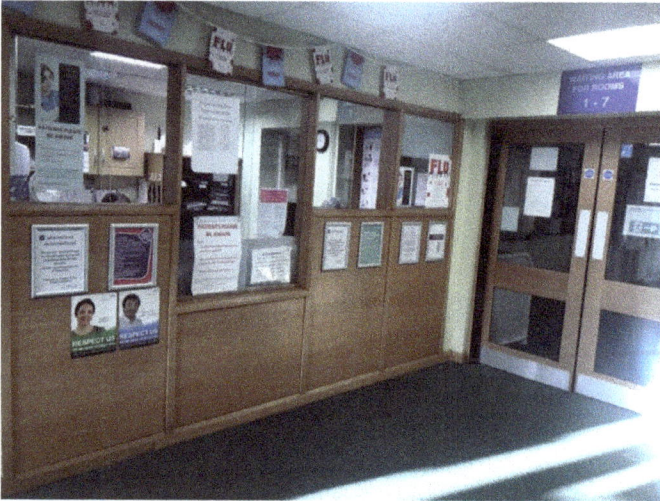

Reception

The doors to the right of reception lead to the main waiting room.

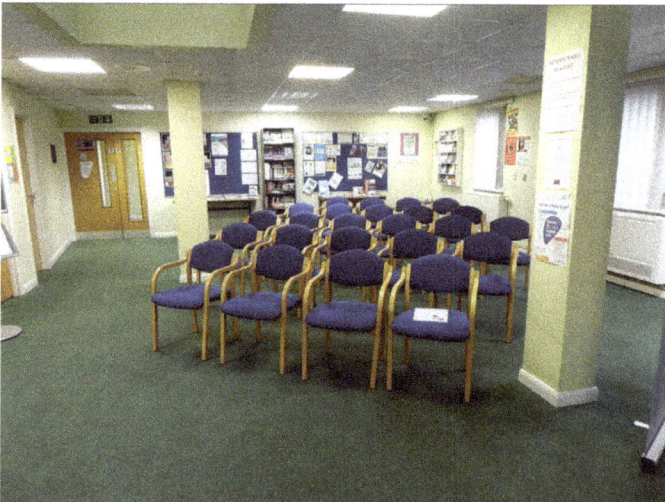

The waiting room

The door at the end of the waiting room on the left leads to the long corridor.

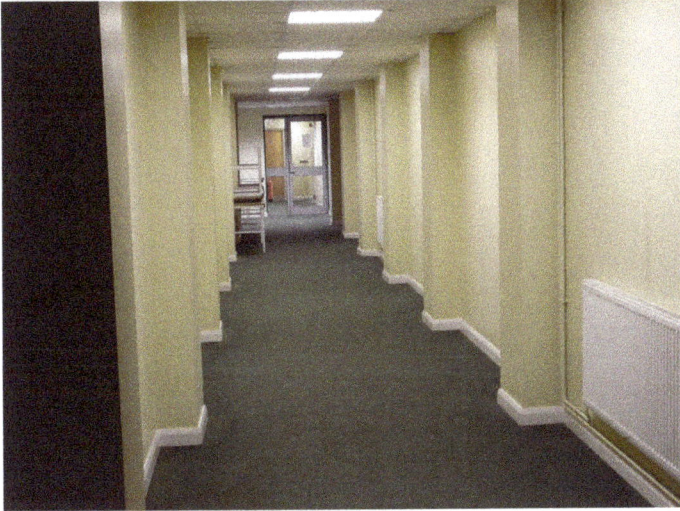

The long corridor.

This corridor leads to a second ground floor waiting room.

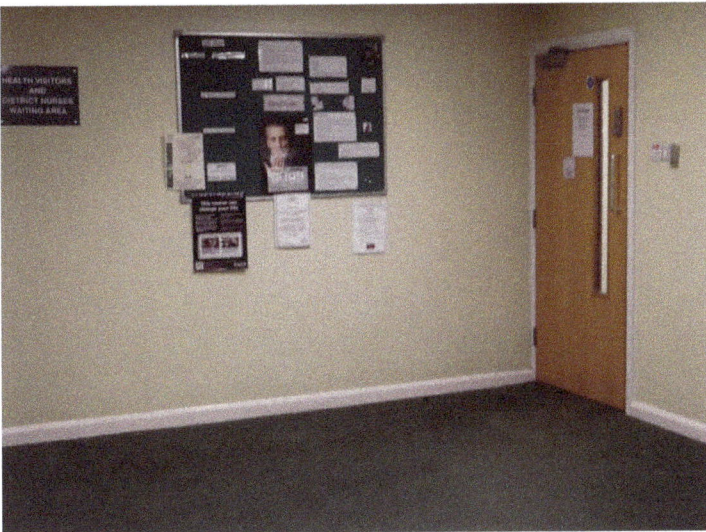

Second waiting room leading to second extension

The door from there leads into what were the two extensions in my garden. These were refurbished in the new build.

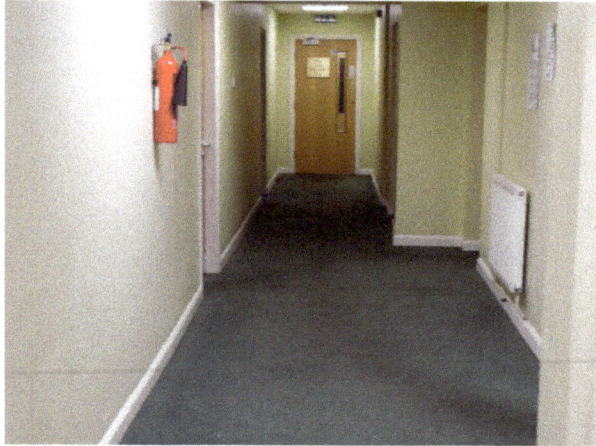

Corridor in second refurbished extension leading to Education Suite

There are numerous rooms in this section of the surgery. Some house district nurses, others health visitors and another staff from the Clinical Commissioning Group's Vanguard workers. A fee is paid to the clinic for use of these rooms. This was so in early 2019, but most of these rooms are now empty in July 2019. It is intended to rent them out again.

The door two-thirds of the way down this corridor is the entrance to The Sloan Education Suite.

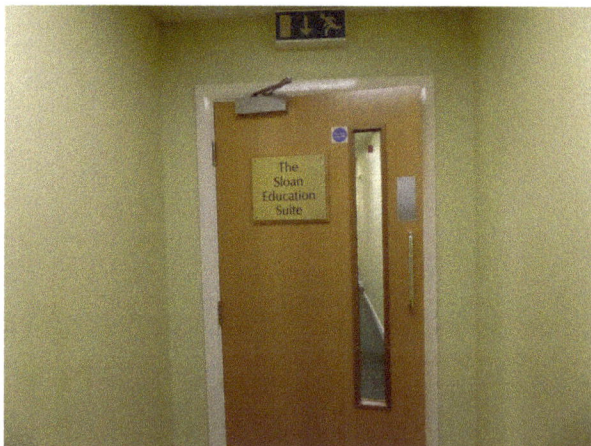

Education suite door

Before I retired, I was allowed to manage the space after this door, but it was not until my leaving event that it was revealed what the area was to be called. I was absolutely thrilled. GP education was the love of my professional life. There are two small meeting rooms, a kitchen, a lavatory, a door to the outside and at the end of that section a large room that can be used as a board room as well as for presentations. I use that room regularly for meetings of a group of retired GPs and locums.

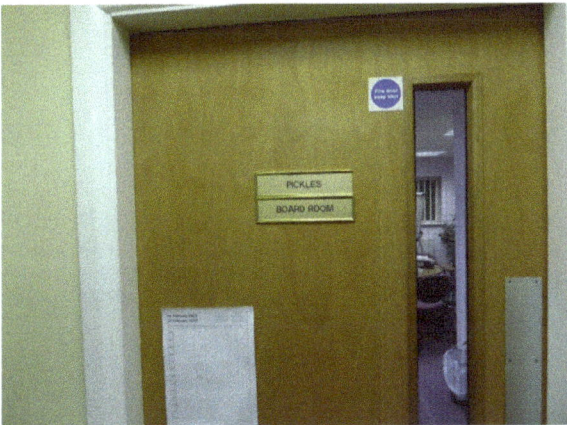

Pickles Board room door

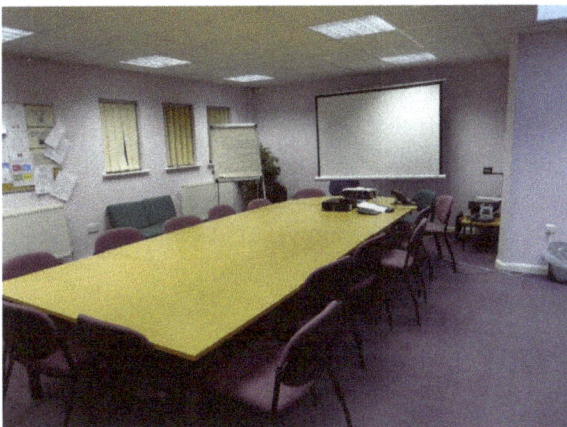

Pickles Board/Training room

William Pickles (1885–1968) was a general practitioner who was the first president of the Royal College of General Practitioners in 1953.

Opposite reception is a lift and stairs leading to two more floors.

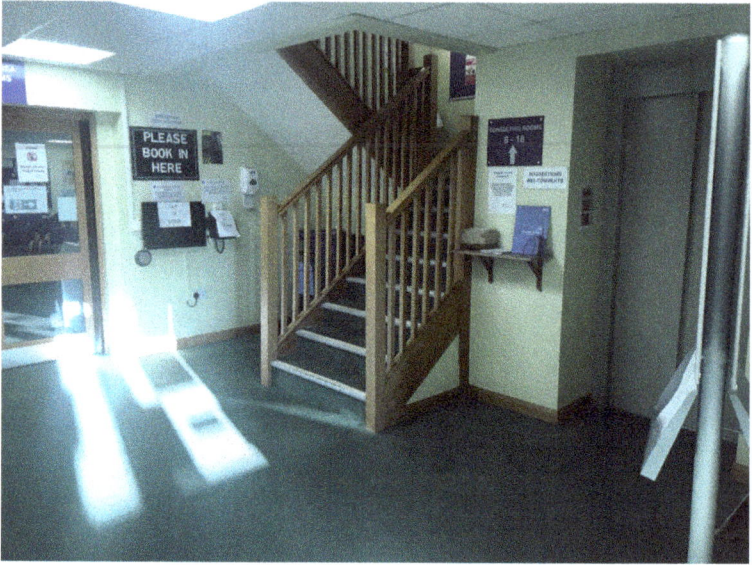

Stairs and lift to first and small second floor

Patients can use the lift to access the first floor only, as the top floor area is for administration and a common room.

There is a third small waiting area for the patients at the top of the stairs to the first floor. The nurses and healthcare assistants work on the first floor and one of the partners had a room there in my time. There are also four consulting rooms which can be used for outside healthcare and other workers.

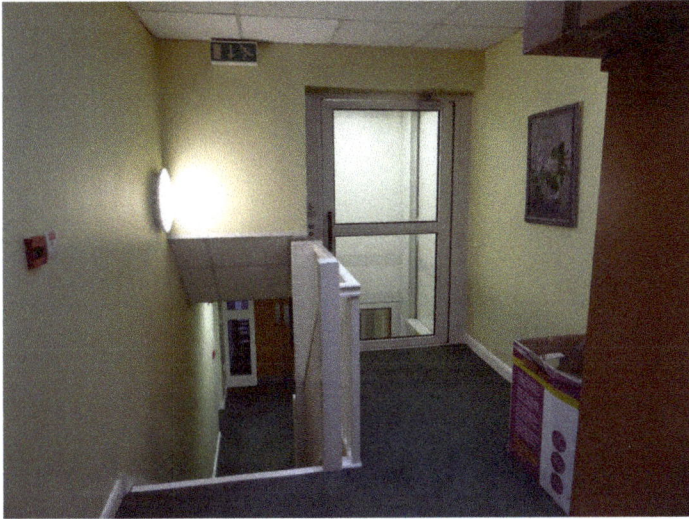

Stairs and lift leading back to first floor

At the top of the stairs, on the second floor is the practice manager's office and another room for administration.

Stairs and a lift for staff lead down to a couple of rooms and a common room. One room is for the secretary and the other for the administrator of prescriptions. The regulations stipulated that we had to have a lift for disabled staff. We were planning a Stannah Stairlift. After a building inspection, we were told that we were not allowed to have such a lift because of health and safety issues. To meet the regulations, we had to spend £10,000 on the lift which is on the right. I had some evil thoughts about that lift. The evil thought of mine was that I was going to break a receptionist's leg so that the expenditure was worthwhile. The sad thing was that after that bad thought, Carolyn Cranton broke her ankle and had to use that lift. Thank you, Carolyn. It was all worthwhile after all.

The common room at the end of the building is entered after the two rooms described above.

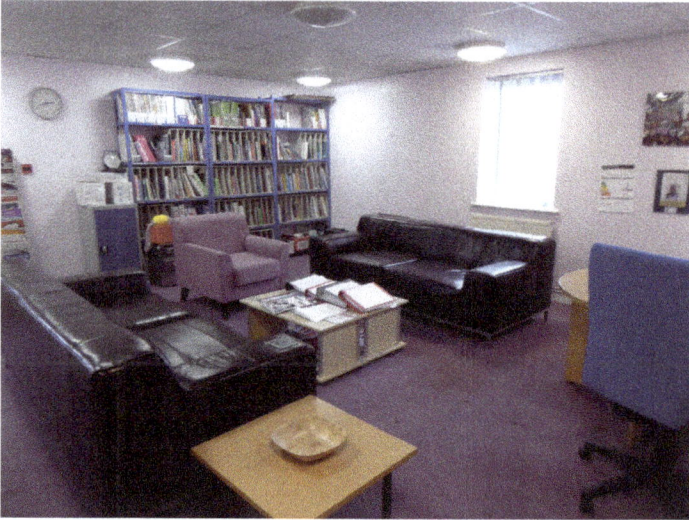

Common room showing library

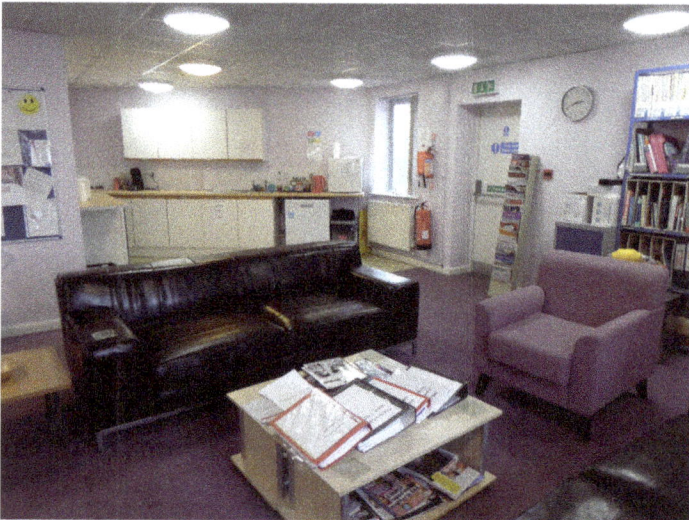

Common room showing kitchen area

To the left of the kitchen area is a door leading to two lavatories. There is a fire exit door on the right with metal steps leading to the car park outside. This door has mainly been used for Lynn to get outside to have a fag. The common room is a great luxury where one can escape and relax for a short time.

The above tour of the new medical centre requires some concentration to visualise it.

Tieve Tara Medical Centre was officially opened jointly by Yvette Cooper MP and Maureen Wood. (See photos and explanation in the chapter on cleaners.)

* * *

The rooms of the old surgery were used for all sorts of things by my parents and me. The waiting room was used for my birthday parties. In 1951 my sixth birthday was held there. My mother had seen an advert for Harry Corbett and Sooty and hired them. The only photo I have of the old waiting room is the one of Sooty. The photo was taken by Jack Hulme who became a famous photographer (see chapter on patients).

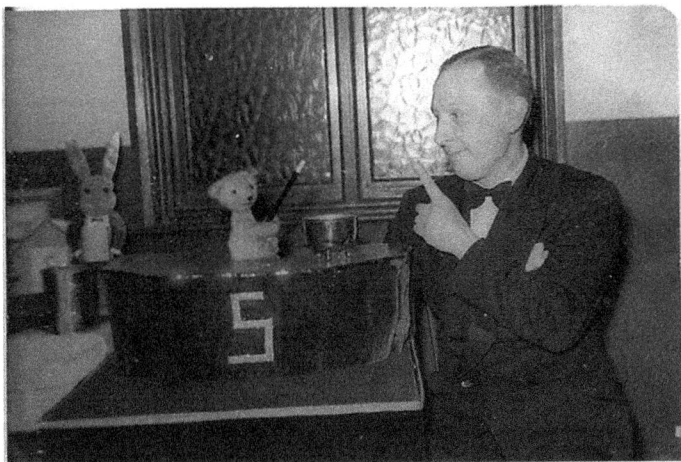

Harry Corbett and Sooty. Photo by Jack Hulme.

In 2018 I was asked to write blogs for NHS England and the National Association of Primary Care (NAPC). This was part of the celebration of the seventieth anniversary of the foundation of the NHS. The NAPC asked if I had any photos and I sent them this one. They were over the moon as it was Sooty's seventieth birthday that year too. The photo was put on their website.

My twenty-first birthday party was also held in the waiting room. Steve Shalet (mentioned in the introduction) came. My parents had a few friends round and they were in the sitting room. Steve mistakenly went into that room and asked, "Have you any of the hard stuff?" I think I was only allowed cider in the waiting room party. Kath was also at that party.

My longest standing good friend is George Goodenough. My mother organised dancing lessons for us in the old waiting room. I hated these lessons. I think George did as well.

Martin and Jennifer Smith are relations through Kath, and we spent many Christmases with them and their children, either in their house in Leeds or ours. I am not sure how old their children, Claire and Nigel, were when this scenario was played out in the original surgery. I think Nigel was about ten and Claire older. Nigel was the doctor and sat in the main consulting room. Claire was the receptionist. I was the patient and sat in the waiting room. Claire showed me to the doctor and Nigel asked me how I was. I answered that I had been getting headaches. The treatment for that particular complaint was Nigel thumping me in the chest!

There have been one or two criminal incidents with both the house and surgery over the years.

When my mother was working in the old surgery by herself after my father died, she was burgled a number of times. The break-ins were right at the opposite side of the building from her consulting room. Nothing really valuable was stolen. There was never a break-in at night. I think my mother was really brave living alone in that house for so many years.

At one time, in the middle of the night, my parents heard a thumping noise coming from the kitchen. My father kept a lead-tipped truncheon in his bedside table. My father led the way downstairs with my mother close behind with her hand on his shoulder. They quietly entered the kitchen. There was no one there but the dog scratching himself and banging his leg on the kitchen floor. That was Wooffee. I have that truncheon in my bedside table now.

After Kath and I moved in, there were several burglaries, two of which were in the night while we were in bed. It was very frightening indeed. The first was through the kitchen door and all that was stolen was some biscuits and my first attempt at home-made wine. The thief was caught and in his statement he said something like, "I tasted the wine and it was so horrible, I was nearly sick." That upset me more than anything. My diary with all our holidays was stolen on another occasion. The second break-in was into our sitting room and our video recorder was taken. We knew who the thief was each time from patients but there was no evidence. Sales from the burglaries fed a drug habit.

I applied for a grant to provide video cameras for the surgery and house. We were successful and three video cameras were set up. Within a week, the main video camera monitoring the surgery was stolen! Soon after that, I had to explain to someone who had been involved with the awarding of the grant and who wanted to inspect the work.

After each burglary, the insurance company for our house insisted on more and more security measures. The house is like Fort Knox. It now has a monitored burglar alarm, six video cameras with a DVD recorder and a facility for the cameras' views to be seen live from mobile devices. There are also panic alarms. There are bright spotlights round the house that light with sensors when it is dark. The surgery has security fencing and is burglar alarmed.

* * *

I now want to show some photos of the inside of the house and explain the relationships of some of the rooms with the surgery.

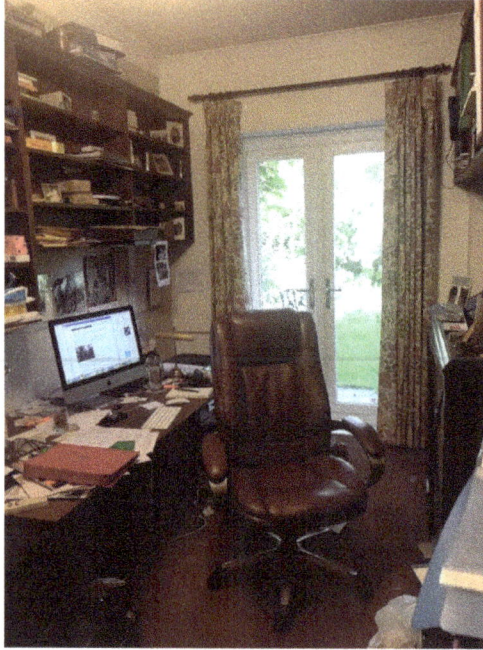

My study

This used to be the dispensary/reception/record-keeping room in the old surgery. It was so when we started in 1978. The wall behind my desk separates the study from an office in the new build.

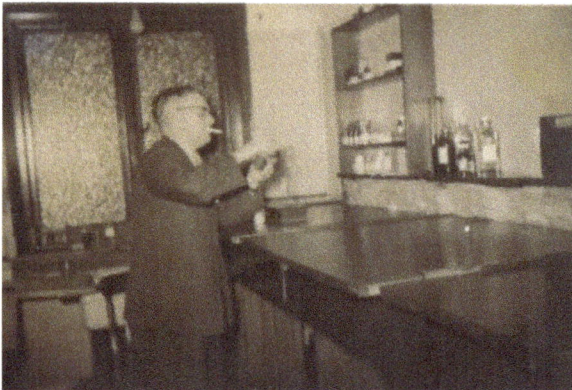

The dispensary and my father

In the above photograph my father, cig on the go, is possibly testing some urine. He is working on one of the wooden covers under which the 10,000 or so patient records were housed. The door to the remainder of the old surgery was blocked off during the first modernisation in the 1980s and that is when we converted that room into my study. The frosted glass windows were replaced with patio doors in 2016. I love my study, especially in the summer with the doors open with sounds of the birds singing and of trickling water from a small fountain.

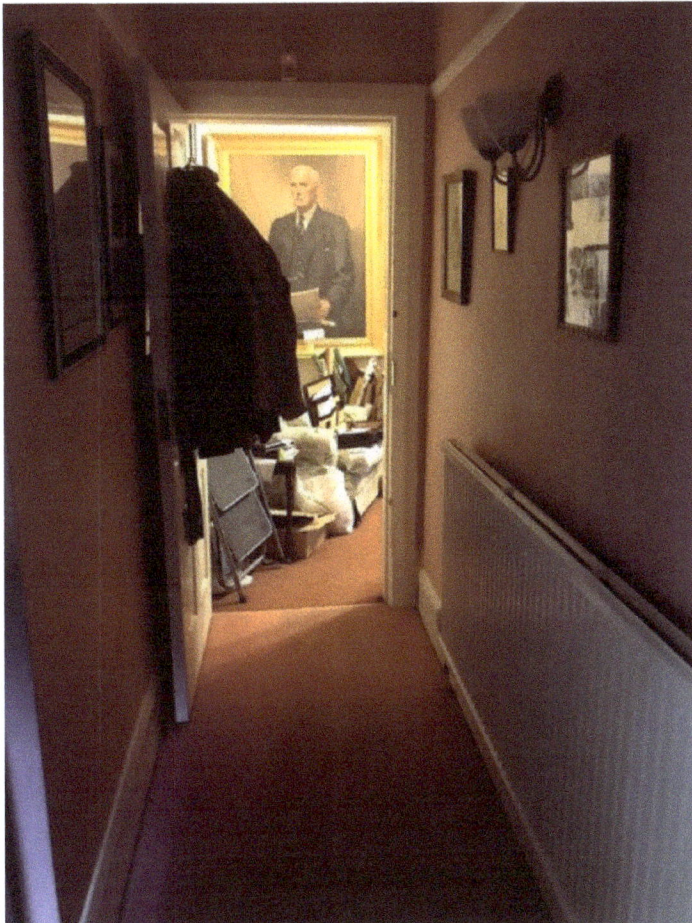

Corridor leading to my study

This door allowed access for my parents to the dispensary but also for the patients to use the lavatory in the house. The portrait is of my paternal grandfather, Francis Sloan. It hangs over the wall where the door from the dispensary to the rest of the old surgery was. It was painted to mark his retirement as headmaster of John's Street School, Lurgan, Northern Ireland in 1935. The name of the street was later changed to Sloan Street.

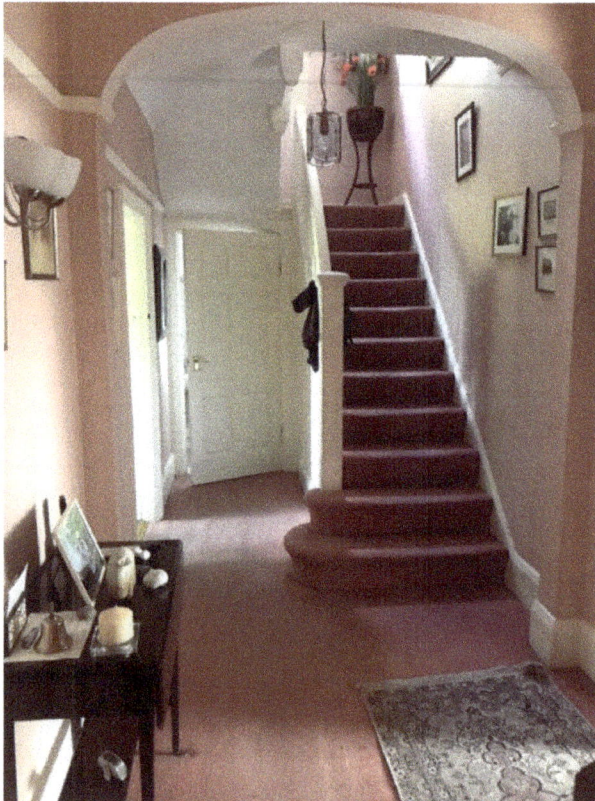

View from door of my study

This view shows the door to the lavatory used by the patients and the family. When I was a kid, I once found a man upstairs wearing a flat cap. He had got lost looking for the lavatory. To the left of the stairs is a door to the kitchen. To the right of the rug is a door to the sitting room.

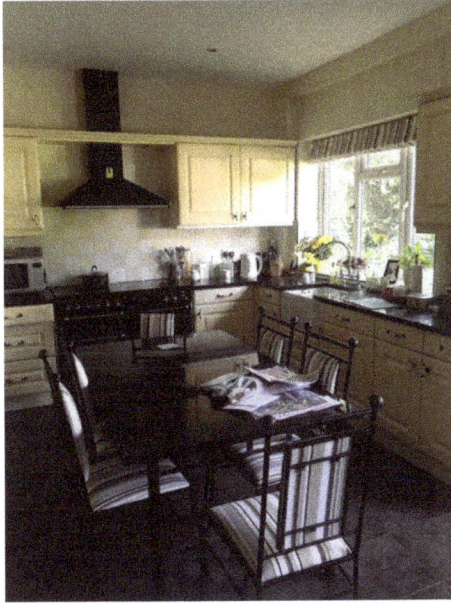

Kitchen

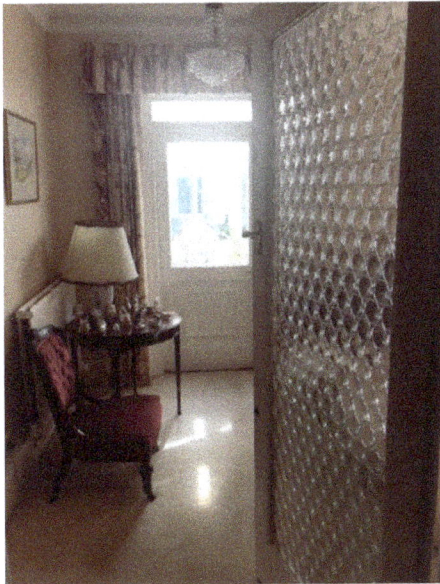

Door to sitting room

This is an original door from when the house was built. The door to the conservatory (added in the 1980s) can be seen.

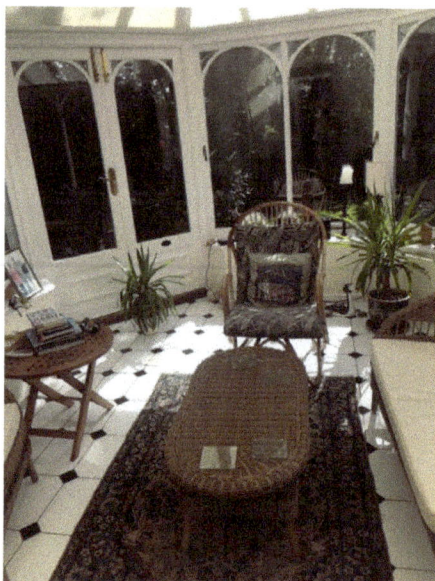

Conservatory, originally the site of the verandah

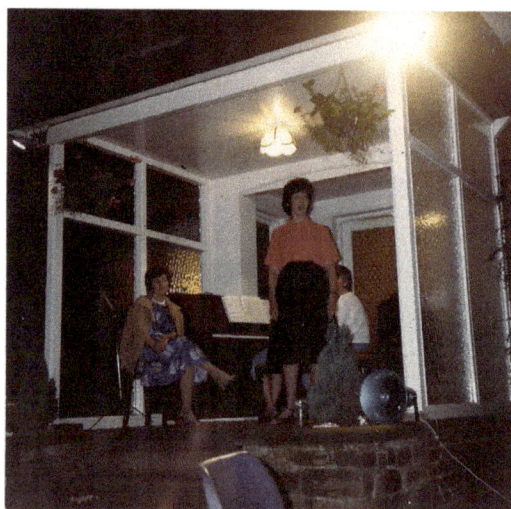

The verandah, mid 1980s

Kath and I held a couple of fundraising events in the house and garden. Kath was heavily involved as a volunteer with the Multiple Sclerosis Society. For a fundraising event for that organisation we dragged the piano from the house to the veranda and Mavis Hunter (singing) and Maureen Chapman, members of the Castleford Choral Society, performed with Kath accompanying.

* * *

The communication systems in the house and surgery have evolved very significantly over the last ninety-plus years. At first there were only landline telephones. Tieve Tara house had bell pushes in downstairs living rooms to call the maid from the kitchen. My live-in nanny, Mrs. Price, answered the telephone and took messages if both my parents were out. They had to phone in to receive the messages. Messages could be also phoned in or left at two other houses in Airedale. When I was a child, we regularly went to the cinema in Castleford on a Thursday afternoon, which was my parents' half day. If their partner was away, the cinematographer would project a message onto the screen in the middle of the film: "Phone call for Dr. Sloan". This was superimposed on the film which continued.

Mobile phones had only been around for a couple of years or so when I started work there in 1978. In the 1980s I bought a pager which I could attach to my belt. I was copying the flash London city businessmen I had seen on the TV. I think the only message I ever received was "don't forget the bread". I phoned home from patients' houses or a phone box (if it had not been vandalised). Reasonable-sized mobile phones took over and were a godsend. However, they too had disadvantages. I was on call one Saturday morning and was in a queue at the post office. I answered a call and the patient wanted to discuss his piles.

Nearly all GPs in the Wakefield district undertook out-of-hours work for a deputising service. It was managed by a group of local GPs. It was a very successful cooperative. I enjoyed working for the cooperative most of the time, as one met doctors one knew. The Coop (as we called it) later owned its own cars. It was great to be driven between visits. There was a fax machine on the back seat which received the details of the visit requests. It was a friendly way to work. I know one of the drivers now who attends my church.

I have always been interested in IT and have kept up with developments. When I was single handed in the early 1980s, the practice bought an Amstrad computer. It cost around £3000 and used floppy discs. I had published a paper in the Journal of the Royal College of General Practice in 1977 on the cost and benefits of practices having an age–sex register of patients. I wanted to make a computerised version. We just managed to fit the 3500 patients' names, addresses and dates of birth on the hard drive. Ann Long, the receptionist, did most of the input. However, I made a terrible error and accidentally erased about 1000 records. In 1987 when two companies, VAMP and Meditel, offered free computers to general practices, the use of computers really took off. Medical records were made on the computer and prescriptions could be typed out. The computer printing of the repeat prescriptions was a great time saver. I spent a lot of evenings in my consulting room writing a programme that was used to help us achieve the childhood vaccination targets. The old records had to be computerised and summaries made.

A year or so before I retired (2005), we changed to the EMIS computer software. In 2008 System One was the software that was preferred by the NHS. This allowed the sharing of clinical data between those members of the NHS family. Let me give you a personal example of this. I developed a complex problem in my right foot in about 2014. I had an MRI scan privately. I was referred to an NHS specialist podiatrist in Normanton. She could get that scan on her computer. Investigation results were sent though daily from the various laboratories and the X-ray department. One had to check these first thing each day and label them as normal etc.

I became a patient of Tieve Tara Medical Centre in 2019. One can make an appointment and order repeat prescriptions online. One can phone in and have a telephone consultation later in the day. I had an appointment with one of the GPs and she made a follow-up appointment there and then. I received an immediate text to my mobile phone as confirmation.

I could have written a whole chapter on the use of IT in general practice. There are a significant number of patients in the area who are not at all familiar with IT and at this time that means getting to the right person for help is difficult. However, I think that IT is the most significant development in the NHS since its birth. It is rapidly developing at present.

* * *

I have lived in the house from 1945 to 1962 and again from 1978 until the time of writing, a total of fifty-seven years. On the whole it has been a very happy place to live and I have very warm memories of my life here: my life with my loving parents and then another life here with my fantastic wife. My mother lived alone in this house for about twenty years after my father died. She coped amazingly well and is a model for my life alone here in Hill House née Tieve Tara.

Chapter 2 – Family

This chapter describes the family members who lived in Tieve Tara/Hill House: my parents, wife, brother and sisters and, of course, our dogs.

My mother, Gerda Laura Clara Alice Sloan, née. Friedmann (1912–1990)

To have photos right back to about 1860 is somewhat rare so I have taken the opportunity of setting them out in this publication.

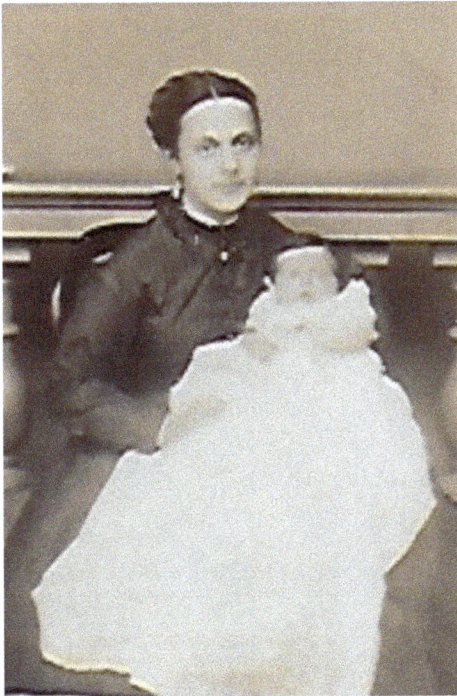

Laura Schlesinger-Trier 1848-1936 (my great great grandmother) with Alice Speyer (my great grandmother) on her knee.

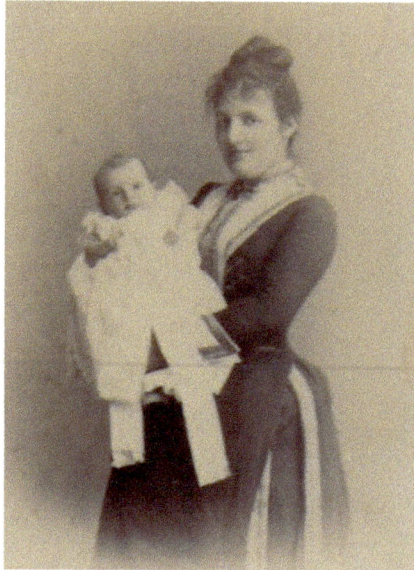

Alice Speyer 1867-1926 (my great grandmother)
holding Lilly Friedmann (my grandmother).

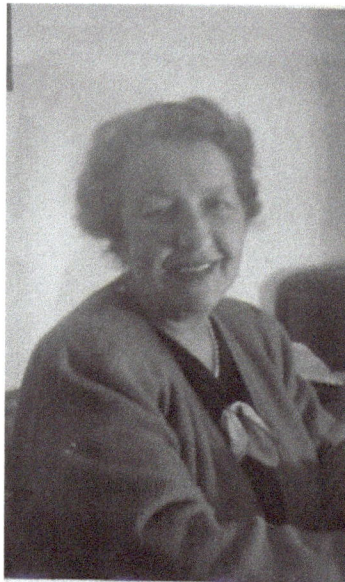

Lilly Friedmann (my grandmother) 1889-1952

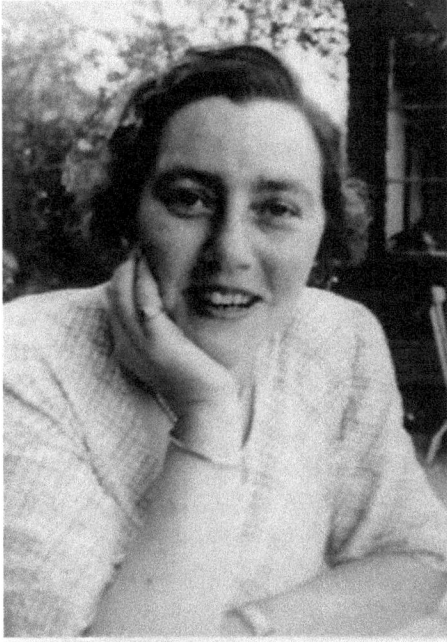

Gerda Sloan

My mother was born in Berlin in 1912 and her parents, Richard and Lilly, were very wealthy and Jewish. I think it is important to briefly describe her lifestyle as she grew up in Berlin to show the contrast with her life in Castleford, England.

Her father, Richard Leopold, was a lawyer (a doctor of law). I am called after him. My mother told me that to understand my grandfather's status I should think of his being the German equivalent of Lord Arnold Goodman, who was a Jewish lawyer and political advisor in London.

My mother and her brothers, Herbert and Ernst, started their education with a live-in English governess, Miss Henderson. They each spoke excellent English at a very early age. I believe they could speak English better than German when they were very young. Their house in Berlin was huge and furnished with antiques and with significant works of art. They often holidayed in Monte Carlo, where my grandfather could play roulette and poker. He owned racehorses, and my mother was an accomplished rider. At one time he also owned a film starring Richard Tauber, the tenor, with whom he was a friend. The film was a flop. My grandfather had someone visit the house to shave him each morning. They had lavish dinner parties and I possess the table plans and menus from some of these. At one point he owned a telephone factory and installed the telephones in the Vatican. A Pope died soon after the phones were up and running. There is a family joke that the Pope, when he felt terribly ill, could not reach the phone on his bedside table and that this resulted in his death.

My mother had a good education and studied medicine at the University of Berlin. Hitler rose to power, and she and some of her friends had to wear yellow armbands at medical school because they were of the Jewish race. However, my grandparents and their children were brought up worshipping in the Lutheran church. I am not sure my mother had ever been in a synagogue. I have only been into a synagogue service once and that was to my friend Steve (see acknowledgements) and Carol's wedding. I am Jewish and became a Catholic in 2016. My late wife became a Catholic in 2006.

You will see in the chapter about my father that there are twenty-two doctors on his side of the family. These were mainly general practitioners. On my mother's side there are some famous medical scientists and one music maker.

Professor Carl Prausnitz (1876–1963) was an internationally famous bacteriologist. He was the father of Otto, who married my mother's cousin, Yella. Carl's father, also called Otto, was a physician. Otto, the father, married an English woman whose surname was Giles. Carl moved to the UK in 1933 and called himself Prausnitz-Giles. After some time working in science laboratories, he became a general practitioner on the Isle of Wight. He changed his surname to Giles. He was a kind and compassionate man and was known there as Father Giles. He continued working as a GP there well into his eighties. When he was 83, he climbed to the top of Simbolica Dam with his medical bag to attend to an injured holidaymaker.

Professor Ernst Joseph Friedmann (1877–1956) was my grandfather's brother so was my mother's uncle. He too was internationally famous and was a biochemist. He managed to leave Germany and became a professor of biochemistry at Cambridge University. He is remembered now because he was the first person to discover the chemical structure of a hormone. He published the chemical formula of adrenaline (then called epinephrine) in 1906. I was thrilled that he was mentioned in one of my biochemistry textbooks when I was a medical student. One of my mother's two brothers was called Ernst and one of my middle names is Ernest.

My mother's Tante (Aunt) Margot was married to Alfred Friedmann, another of my grandfather Richard's four brothers. Margot's maiden name was Neisser. I knew her well when I was a child and then a student and young doctor in London. I met her quite a lot and liked her very much. She spoke seven languages. She was the granddaughter of Professor Albert Ludwig Sigesmund Neisser (1855–1916). He is seriously famous. He discovered the bacterium that caused gonorrhoea and it was called after him (Neisseria gonorrhoeae). He also discovered the causative agent of leprosy.

Perhaps our most famous relation on my mother's side is Felix Mendelssohn-Bartholdy, the composer. The music maker. My grandmother's cousin, Edith, married Ludwig, Mendelssohn's grandson. I was intrigued by this relationship when I was a teenager. At that time Edith was in her eighties and fronted a German TV programme for the elderly. My mother contacted her, and Edith wrote to me accompanied by a photograph of a painting of Felix which she assured me was a true likeness. I have kept Edith's letter to this day and the framed picture of "Uncle" Felix is on the wall next to my piano.

My grandfather had significant business interests in England. He became a naturalised citizen of Great Britain in 1933, as did Lilly, his wife. They emigrated to London that year. They had a flat in Maida Vale in London. They moved to an apartment in Harrogate for the duration of the Second World War and afterwards back to London. He could not afford to insure his valuables. (I have an inventory of those which he sold in England.) He stored half of the larger items in Berlin and the other half in

London. English bombing destroyed the former and German bombs the latter.

My mother was determined to complete her medical studies and obtained her Doctor of Medicine (MD) in 1938. She left Germany immediately after qualifying and only just escaped the country in time to save her life. The British Government announced that foreign doctors had to qualify again by re-taking the final examination. She passed the conjoint finals (MRCS, LRCP) in Edinburgh. I thought that was very impressive. Shortly after passing those exams, the government announced that there was no longer any need for German doctors to retake those exams!

She applied for about three hundred jobs and got nowhere. My father (who was at that time a general practitioner living in Tieve Tara) was in the middle of a very difficult divorce and had advertised for an assistant. He read my mother's application and said to a friend, "I only hope she is not good looking." They were married in 1944! Nearly one year later (more than nine months), I was born.

For the duration of the war, my mother was under a curfew and was not allowed out in the evenings or at night. A policeman would check on her every evening and joined my parents for a relaxing cup of tea. My mother thought this was a great luxury for a GP – not to be allowed out at night. My father must have done all the night visits.

I was born in Dennison Hall Nursing Home, Leeds. There was no NHS at that time, and I was a private birth. My father was so happy after the birth that he put a roll of five pound notes in an empty Elastoplast tin and gave it to the consultant obstetrician. My mother had difficulty sleeping and was given chloral hydrate in liquid form. It tasted very strong and as she was sinking into a deep sleep, she told a nurse that it was the wrong dose. They had accidentally made the medication up to a great strength and she had to have a stomach washout. I suppose these days that would have resulted in a complaint. I often say that my mother had to have a stomach washout as a result of my birth. She stopped smoking cigarettes (Players Weights) when she was thirty-eight weeks pregnant. She never smoked again. I told her that if she had stopped smoking before she became pregnant, I would have been really brainy.

My father asked a patient if she would become a live-in nanny. She was called Mrs. Price and I called her Ninnie. She was over 70 and had been a wet nurse in her early life. (A wet nurse breastfeeds another's child.) She had osteoarthritis and was overweight and my father thought she would not live for long. These two conditions resulted in her having to come downstairs backwards, which amused me a lot as a child. She had her own bedroom and her own sitting room where my toys were. She ate her meals in that room and she had a TV.

My mother only had three weeks off work after I was born. Employing Mrs. Price enabled her to work full time. Mrs. Price took phone messages when both my parents were out. I was sometimes pretty naughty and used to go upstairs and make the telephone bell tinkle by rapidly moving the receiver rests. I could hear her shouting, "I'm coming. I'm coming." She could not move fast because of the arthritis. I also used to tell her to hurry up when I was walking behind her.

Every Sunday she would go into town and visit her daughter, Maud. My father arranged that Norman Dean, the undertaker, took her there and back in one of his limousines.

Mrs. Price was superstitious about thunderstorms. At the onset of a storm, she would put any metal things under a table and these included cutlery. It took her such a long time that the storm has usually finished before the metal objects were all hidden. My father's skills at judging her longevity were not at all good. I left home to go to university and came back for her ninetieth birthday. My mother would take her breakfast in bed and I think a point came when she had to stay upstairs. Her grandson, Mr. Merry, was a patient of mine whom I meet occasionally now when I am in Castleford town. Mrs. Price died not long after her ninetieth birthday. That age was regarded as very old in those days.

What always amazed me was how the people of Airedale and Castleford took to my mother, a German, in the middle of the Second World War. She, at the same time, took to the people of Airedale and was always grateful for their giving her such a warm welcome. This was because she was a refugee but also because she was so kind and caring to her patients. She was so thankful that Great Britain took her in and let her do the job of her dreams. Their housekeeper, Mrs. McGrath, had a son, Harry, who was a prisoner of war in Germany in that war and contracted TB there. He eventually died as a result of that disease in the early 1960s. I don't think Harry ever had an ill thought about my mother. Indeed, he used to drive her or my father occasionally.

My mother was a modern woman. She was the first woman in Castleford to wear trousers (slacks). She was a cultured woman and took us to the ballet, concerts and musicals in London, and she read widely. She was a good bridge player and liked to bet on the horses. She loved travelling and went to Jerusalem on her own after my father died. She was always rather naughty, and she sent me a postcard telling me she had had a ham sandwich there. Jews don't eat pork and ham.

I saw how the war affected my mother for the rest of her life. She had problems sleeping and, like she did in the war, listened to the news half the night on the BBC World Service. She knew that if Hitler had won that she was on a death list. She had a serious guilt complex that she had survived and had not died in a concentration camp. There is a known condition called survivor guilt. Her mother's cousin Peter Speyer died in Auschwitz in 1943. I think I know to an extent what it must feel like to have to leave one's country and become a refugee.

My mother's parents moved back to London after the war ended. In 1952 her father died suddenly and shortly afterwards her mother, Lilly, committed suicide by cutting her wrists in the bath. I was 7 years old. I think they told me they had both died, but I really can't remember. I wonder if this was psychological repression. My paternal grandfather died about that time also and they did not tell me about that for a year. I cannot remember either of my parents being at all upset and my happy childhood simply continued. Lilly, like my mother, was a very loving person. My mother's father was a gambler, drinker and womaniser. He was a character and I loved hearing the stories about him. We will never know why Lilly committed suicide.

This selfish act of my grandmother had a considerable effect on my mother, magnified by the fact that one of her brothers, Ernst, blamed her for not getting to her mother in London quickly enough after her father's death. This added to her already significant guilt complex as a survivor of the war. She drank too much alcohol but mainly in the evenings. The drinking did not affect her job in the daytime. My father was a teetotaller!! She developed oesophageal varices and had cirrhosis of the liver when she died in 1990 aged 77. I regret the rows we had in her later life about her excessive drinking. I wanted her to be well and loved her. I forgave my mother everything because she deeply loved my father, her mother and me. I put her death certificate in my drinks cabinet for a while! It is not in there now.

My mother was a very loving and generous person. I cannot remember her being anything but kind and loving towards me. She always supported me, as did my father. I was petrified that my mother would commit suicide after my father's death. They bought me a car when I became a student in 1963 and my mother bought me two further cars later. In 1970 when Felicity and I married, she gave us a house she owned in Airedale. This was a wedding gift. Like most Jewish people, she was astute when it came to money. There was a significant tax advantage to giving us that house. However, that does not detract from her generosity.

When I got a job as a GP in Cheltenham, my mother moved down there to be near me. I sold the house in Airedale and it funded the purchase of a flat in Budleigh Salterton owned by my friend Bill Bullingham's brother, Chris. Bill bought the Airedale House without even seeing it. Bill and I did have a business arrangement for if he sold it badly. The sale of that flat funded my second wife, Kath, and I setting up the general practice from scratch in Airedale, Castleford, after my mother had retired. Tieve Tara house and surgery were empty during that time.

Building up the practice from a base with no patients was very difficult. Of course, all my new patients had to come from neighbouring practices. At one point my mother broke her agreement with her former partner not to practice again in Castleford for five years after retirement. She helped me out when I was under great stress. She actually became my medical partner for over a year. Consequently, her former partner served an injunction on her and we had to close the practice for a few days. My mother would be proud that Kath and I built up a thriving training practice which won awards and ended up with a huge building with nineteen consulting rooms. After the initial build up, Kath did another couple of jobs and then became the practice manager until 2000. Kath and my parents are commemorated on the Foundation Wall of the Royal College of General Practitioners.

My mother's dogs

The first dog was bought for me and I named him Wooffee (spelled double-U, double O, double F, double E). He was a Welsh Terrier.

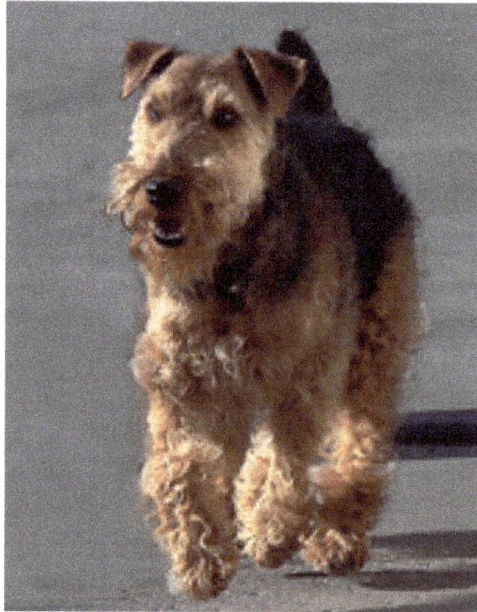

Welsh Terrier

He was not very well behaved. My Aunty Agnes from Wakefield called him "Scruffy". My mother used to beckon him with chocolate such that he thought he was called Chocolate.

42

Next door to our house is a magnesian limestone quarry. He fell down that once and broke his leg. He was lucky to survive. He once spent the night on my bed with me and bit my big toe and made it bleed. My mother used to take him out with her on her house calls. One of her cars was a Hillman Minx drophead coupé. When the roof was down, Wooffee would be on the back seat with his lead tied to the struts of the roof. One day, as she was driving, he jumped out of the back and was hanging by his lead with his back paws scraping the road. Pedestrians were pointing animately at the car as she passed. My mother thought they were patients waving and she waved back until she realised something was amiss. Wooffee survived that one as well. He did not really like cars leaving the house and would bite a back tyre as a car was setting off.

Nearly every Sunday afternoon, we would get together with the Goodenoughs, close family friends. We might go to their house two miles away in Castleford or they would come to ours. Often, when they had left our house and were well on their way home, Wooffee would run the two miles and find their house. He must have done that by smell as they arrived home before he set off. I was told recently by Alan Goodenough that Wooffee arrrived very thirsty and would drink out of their grandfather's spittoon. Wooffee was sometimes badly behaved. My mother had read in a medical journal that Librium (chlordiazepoxide) was used in stun guns to knock tigers out. (Librium is in the same class of drugs as Valium.) She gave Wooffee a 5 mg capsule. I remember him walking – or rather sliding – along a wall with a very glazed look. She did not give him that drug again.

Her next three dogs were Regie, Tovi and Puppie. Regie (called after me – R E G Sloan) was a Miniature Schnauzer. The other two after Regie were Yorkshire Terriers.

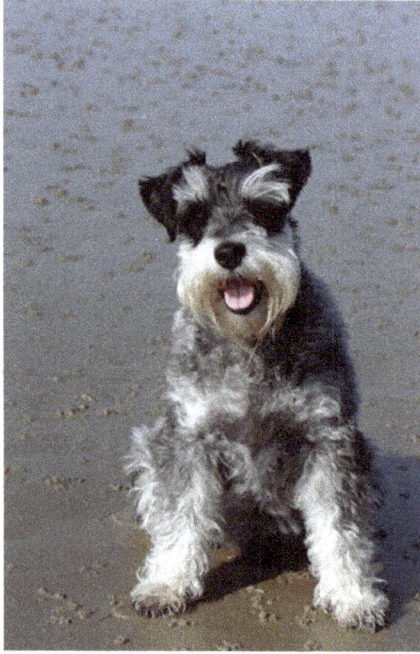

Miniature Schnauzer

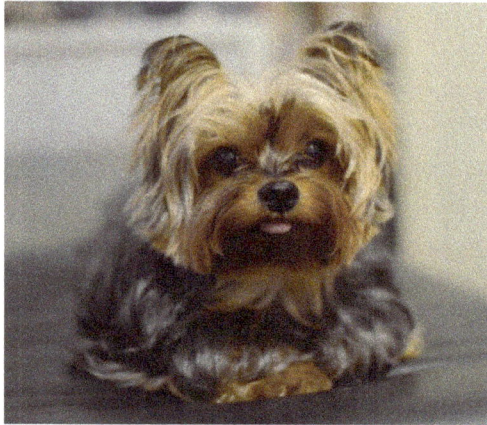

Yorkshire Terrier

When my mother was a child, the family dog was a Pekingese. It was called Changie.

I possess what I think is something unique, which I will describe to you in the photos that follow.

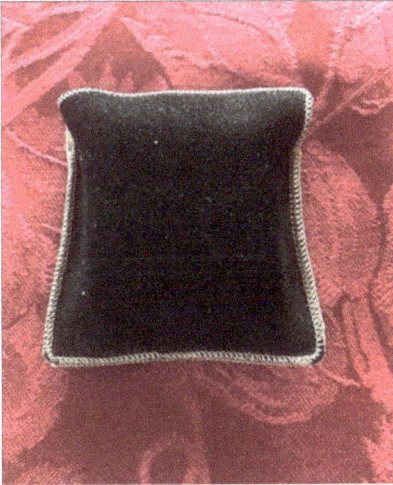

A black velevet pouch

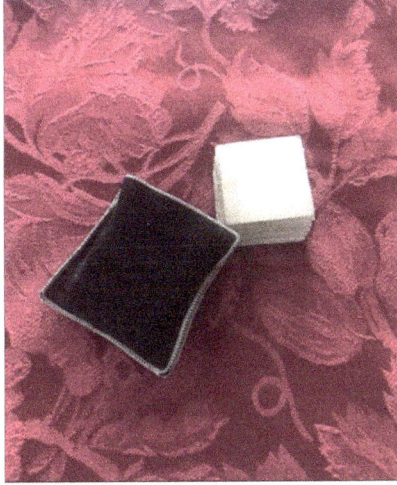

containing concertinaed photos

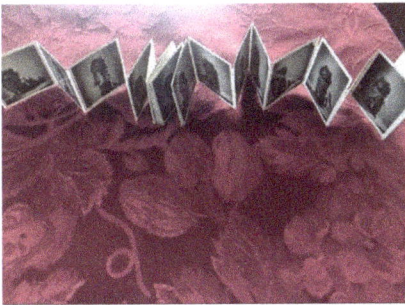

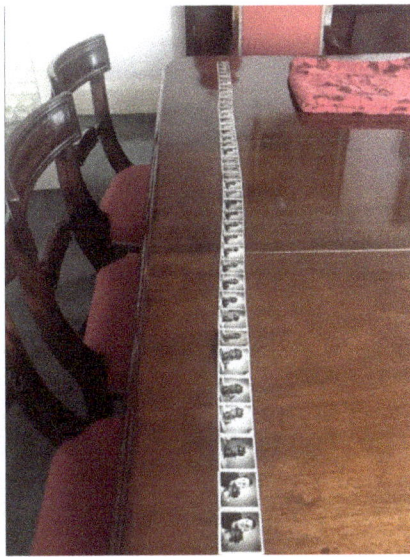

43 photos of a Pekingese including 2 sets of my mother with the dog

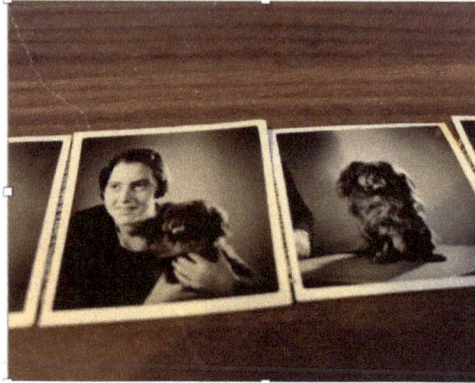

The dog might not be Changie. I think it was my grandmother's after they came to England.

Towards the end of her general practice working life, my mother was in the habit of having Regie in her consulting room during a surgery. He used to settle down on a towel on the examination couch!

After my father died, my mother's dogs were company and a major part in her life. She lived alone from 1966 to 1990 but led a full life with friends, playing bridge, betting on the horses, etc. She continued going on holiday. As I mention in another chapter, she holidayed often with her friend Edna Box, the then retired practice midwife.

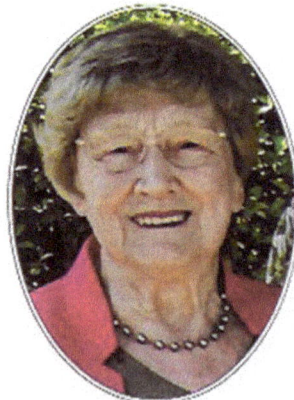

Edna Clarice Box in 2018

I have learned a lot from my mother and others about how to cope with bereavement and living alone. Towards the end of her life, I sat with her in her nursing home. She could not communicate. On the TV in her room, footage was being shown of the Berlin Wall coming down. How she would have loved to see that momentous event.

Her ashes were buried in a joint grave with my father's in Putney Vale Cemetery, London. Her parents' ashes are in the adjacent grave. It was at the request of my father that his ashes were buried next to his in-laws so that in the end my mother's ashes could be near his and her parents'.

My father, George Thomas Wake Sloan (1898–1967)

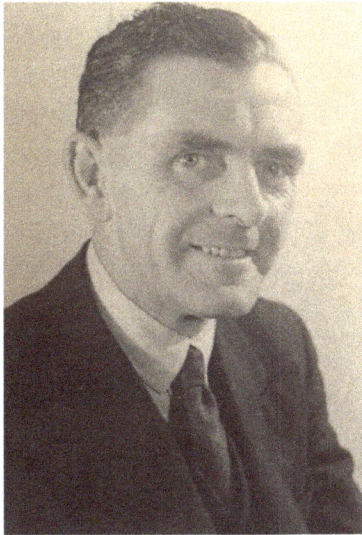

George Sloan

My father was born in Lurgan, Northern Ireland, in 1898. His father was called Francis and was a headmaster of John's Street Primary School in that town. His mother was called Georgina Sarah Wake. There are five relations in his family tree called Thomas.

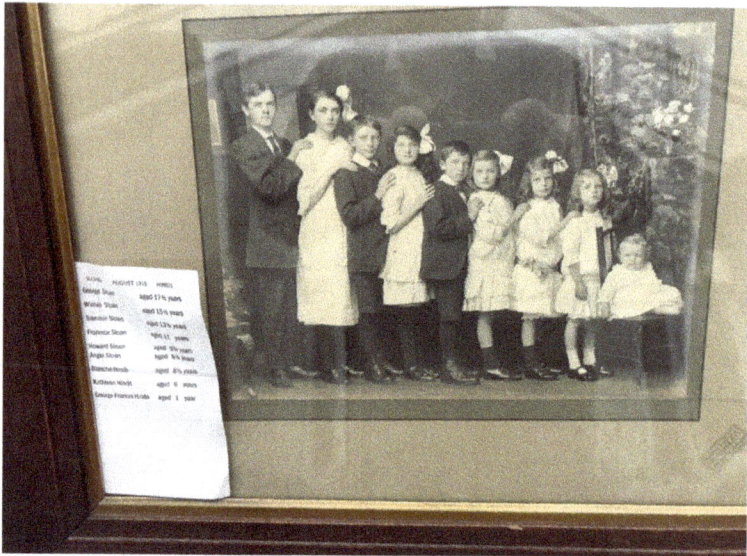

The Sloan family c 1915

In the picture of the Sloan family, my father is the eldest on the left, followed by his five siblings and three cousins. All three men went to Queen's University Belfast to study medicine. My grandmother worked her fingers to the bone taking in knitting etc. to pay for their education. Sadly, the youngest of the brothers, Howard, died from a neurological disease while he was a medical student. The youngest sister, Florence, died in her forties or fifties. I have a book of her poems. The eldest sister, Winnie, obtained a BA in French at Queen's University Belfast and Angel became a dispenser in a pharmacy in that city. My father and his remaining brother, Sam, became general practitioners in Yorkshire, the former in Castleford and the latter in Wakefield, about 10 miles away.

My father was the first doctor in his family. Over the years there have been twenty-two of his family in the medical profession.

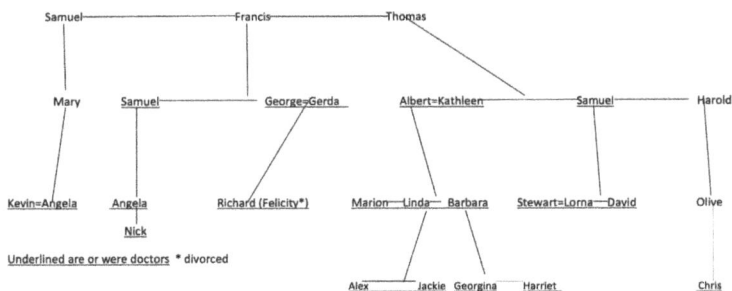

Samuel———————Francis—————Thomas

Mary   Samuel—————George=Gerda   Albert=Kathleen————Samuel————Harold

Kevin=Angela   Angela   Richard (Felicity*)   Marion——Linda— Barbara   Stewart=Lorna—David   Olive

Nick

Underlined are or were doctors * divorced

Alex————Jackie Georgina   Harriet   Chris

21.8 18   22 doctors in the family on father's side

Sloan family tree of doctors

Medical students at Queen's had to undertake their maternity training in Dublin and a special degree was awarded for that as well as the usual degrees in surgery and medicine: the BAO (Bachelor of the Art of Obstetrics). Delivering babies was an art, as was a lot else in medical practice in the early 1920s and beyond.

After qualifying, my father did a surgical hospital job in Blackburn, Lancashire and then started in general practice in Halifax. It was not long until he went into partnership with a GP in Castleford called Dr. Gilfillan. They knew one another as they both were students at Queen's University Belfast. After a while, they fell out and the town was divided into two. They agreed that my father should look after the patients in the suburb of Airedale and Dr. Gilfillan those in Castleford town. There were many fewer residents in Airedale than in Castleford town, which was relatively more affluent. They did not speak for many years, and eventually they discovered that they were both looking after patients living across the "border". They made it up in the early 1960s.

Practicing as a GP in the 1920s and 1930s was very hard and my father made very little money. The people were poor and there was the Great Depression of the 1930s. My father employed a man, Mr. Firth, a collector of fees. My father bought a house for Mr. and Mrs. Firth. It was that house (41 Airedale Road), mentioned above, that my mother later gave as a wedding present.

Mr. Firth was around when I was a child. He was the spitting image of the actor Richard Hearne, who played Mr. Pastry on children's BBC television.

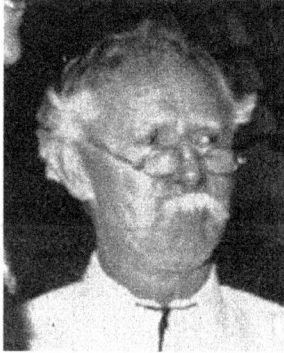

Richard Hearne

Mr. Firth had great trouble extracting money from patients and my father was a very generous and kind person. He let a lot of them off the fees owed. There was significant poverty at that time. The Firths had a son called Eric. My parents paid for Eric to go to medical school, but sadly he never completed the course. Eric was a lovely person.

Because of the Blackburn job, my father enjoyed undertaking minor operations in the surgery and had a general anaesthetic machine dispensing ether.

In the Depression, people could not afford to go to the dentist and my father used to extract teeth. He also occasionally practiced euthanasia on pets to save people the vet fees.

In the 1920s he did post-mortem examinations on his own patients. He used to sing and whistle hymns while he was doing these, and there was always a policeman present. The singing and whistling were a result of an experience with one of the first post-mortems he had performed. It was very quiet and suddenly the body made a single loud gasp for breath. My father jumped out of his skin. This is a well-known response shortly after death.

In the middle of one post-mortem, he discovered that he personally had done something which caused the patient's death.

He did something to the corpse that made the policeman feel sick so that he had to go out of the room for a short while. The post-mortem was rapidly completed and "fatty heart" was written on the death certificate instead of "ruptured uterus".

My father was too young to join up for the forces in the First World War (he tried) and too old for the Second World War. In the Second World War, he was in charge of a single-decker bus equipped to deal with medical emergencies if there was an air raid. Bombs were only dropped once or twice on Castleford when it was mistaken for Leeds. An incendiary bomb landed in the garden during one of these raids and he kept its remnants in his consulting room desk drawer. He was a nervous man and for a while after that he had a hosepipe set up in the house in case of fire. I possess the tin hat he used in the war.

He married Matilda McCaw (known as PiPi) and they had three children, Geraldine, Dorothy and Frank. They divorced in the early 1940s. He dearly loved all four of his children.

Geraldine was the eldest. She and her sister, Dorothy, were sent to Hunmanby Hall Girls School in East Yorkshire. Geraldine (Gerry) met her future husband, Johnny Dunn, in the Second World War when he was in the Air Force. They married in 1945. They settled down in Glasgow, where Johnny's parents lived. They had four children: Elizabeth, Michael, Andrew and David (in descending age order).

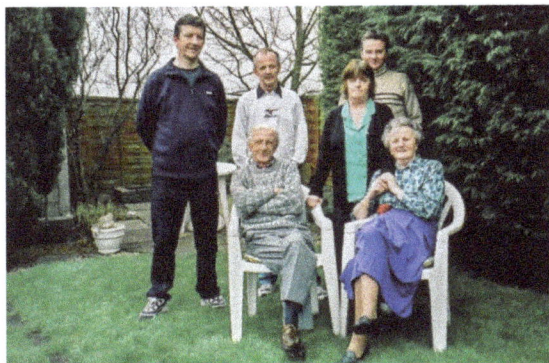

The Dunn's Golden wedding in 1985 (Left to right back – Andrew, Michael, Elizabeth and David. Front – Johnny and Gerry)

Johnny worked with his father mending televisions. I think they started this work in Johnny's parents' garage at their house. They eventually built up a chain of television shops in Glasgow and sold out to the Rank Organisation for a huge amount of money. This was in the early 1960s. As part of the deal, Johnny was offered a directorship of the Rank Organisation. He resigned from this lucrative job because he felt he was doing nothing for them. After making all that money, they moved to a beautiful new house in Rutherglen. It had a tennis court and a lovely garden. They bought a grand piano. Johnny played by ear but mainly only on the black keys. Johnny and Gerry were very generous people. Some of the profit from the sale was spent on buying a house for a friend and some on a butcher's shop for another friend. One time when my parents were staying with them, Johnny and my father were discussing cars. Like me, both of them had a weakness for rather expensive and sometimes fast cars. (Johnny had a Chevrolet Corvette Stingray and he nearly broke my back when I was a passenger as he put his foot down on the accelerator.) He asked my father what the car of his dreams was. My father said it was a Jaguar. Johnny went out of the room and after a while came back with a cheque for the cost of a 2.4 litre model. My father was absolutely thrilled. It was white and like the one the fictional TV detective Inspector Morse drove.

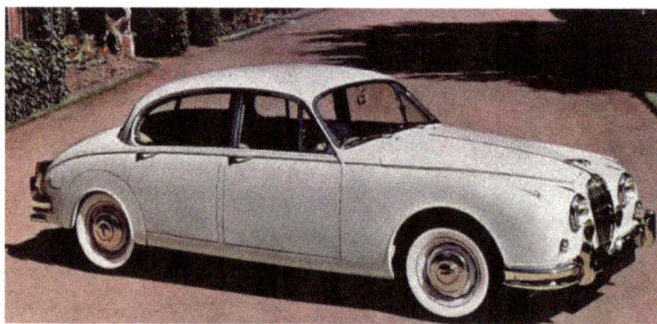

1963 Jaguar saloon

Johnny, Gerry and the family came to stay with us many times when we were young, and we went up to Glasgow and stayed with them. Their daughter Elizabeth is only one year younger than I. I made her call me Uncle Richard. Johnny and Gerry are no longer with us. Their children and I keep in touch to varying degrees. I am Facebook friends with each of them and also with some of Gerry's grandchildren.

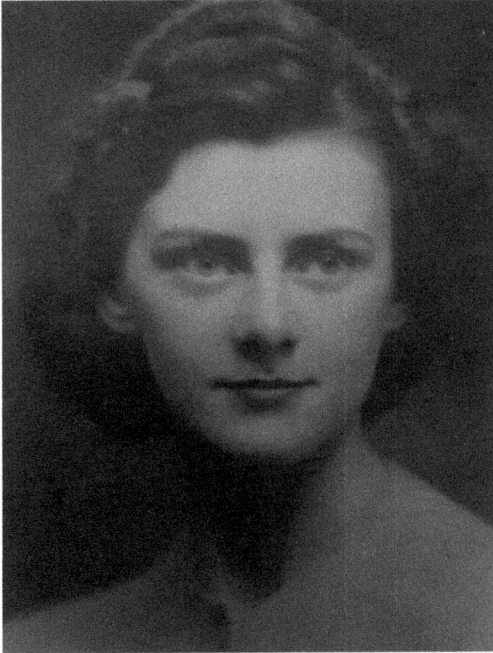

Dorothy (Dot)

Dorothy was the second born and married Derek Fullelove, a Cambridge graduate and a geography teacher. They lived in Africa for a while and then settled in Poulton-le-Fylde, Lancashire. They had three children, all girls. Susan was the eldest and then there were Carol and Helen. Dorothy was a fantastic cook. I have her tomato soup recipe written in her own hand which I use now. She often talked at length and that is a polite way of putting it. I exaggerate only slightly when I say that Kath and I took turns to listen to her. She was a bubbly person. It was a tragedy when she developed dementia at a relatively young age and spent several of her remaining years in a special ward in Blackpool Royal Infirmary.

Derek was fascinated with the pit village of Fryston and the limestone quarry near Tieve Tara. He was a geologist and chipped off samples of the limestone on one visit. He pointed out that Fryston was different from most pit villages. It is virtually in the country and is situated very close to the River Aire. The miners owned horses and also went shooting and fishing.

I keep in touch with Helen. I was one of the trustees for the money Derek left Carol when he died. She was not a well person and she died in 2018.

Frank was only ten years older than me. He lived in Tieve Tara house at the same time as I did but only for a very short time.

He was occasionally badly behaved and was expelled from Silcoates School in Wakefield. I don't know why. The surgery extension to the house had a flat roof. When I was a baby, he put me in a large shopping basket, attached a washing line rope to it and hauled me up. My mother nearly exploded with anger when she found out.

Frank joined the merchant navy when he was 16 years old. He was away from home on his first ship for eighteen months. My father bought a globe to follow his journey. On his first day on that ship, the captain asked the crew if any of them had a relation who was a doctor. My brother was chosen to be the "ship's medical man". He studied to be a radio officer and had to learn Morse code. I used to write him messages in Morse and post them under his bedroom door when he was at home. He eventually became a senior radio officer on P&O cruise ships, which included the Canberra. My parents and I went on a P&O cruise every other year for a while, but we were never on the same ship as Frank.

Frank married Florence, who was brought up in Northern Ireland. She never completed her course as a medical student and eventually worked for Jacob Bronowski when he was director of research at the National Coal Board.

Their first home was in Fareham, near Portsmouth. Frank retired from the merchant navy because of depression and anxiety. They and the children, Christopher and Mary, eventually lived in a lovely house in Northern Ireland. It was in Co. Londonderry near the small town of Limavady. Florence's sister lived next door.

Here follows a fairy story. When their son, Christopher, was a teenager, he befriended Uncle Mervyn. Mervyn lived on his own. Christopher did lots for him. When Mervyn died, he left Christopher a Georgian mansion with 200 acres of farmland and also lots of valuables. Christopher went to university in England and Frank and Florence moved in to and looked after Drumcovitt House. They developed some buildings into self-catering cottages and the farmland was rented out.

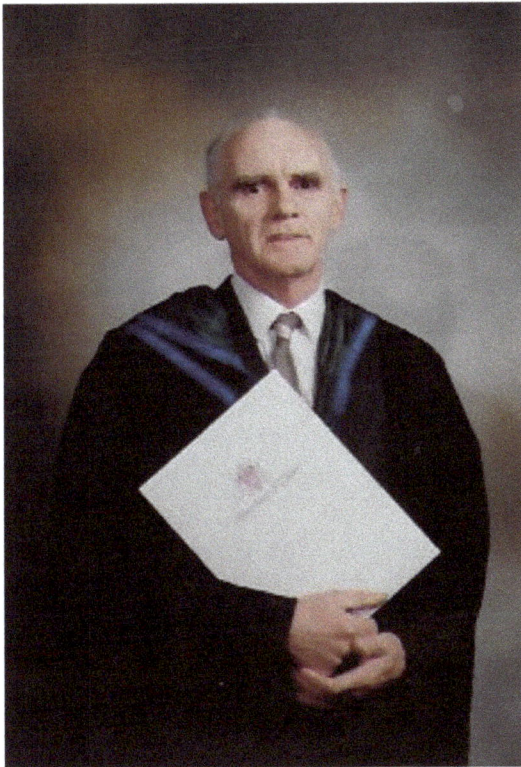

Frank. BA (Hons). Degree ceremony 1994.

Frank and Florence moved out to a bungalow they owned in Limavady when Christopher and his partner Sarah moved in. Sarah manages the holiday cottages (https://drumcovitt.com).

Frank died from lung cancer when he was 71. Before he died, he phoned me and asked me to contact his consultant to ask her to stop going on about his smoking. She was charming and respected the request. Florence died in 2019. She had deep dementia. When I was last over in Northern Ireland, about four years ago, I spent a day with their daughter, Mary, and she took me to where Game of Thrones is filmed. (I am a fan of that programme.) We had a great day together. I am really fond of Christopher and Mary.

* * *

1948 was payoff time for my parents. The National Health Service was formed. Most local consultants and GPs were against the new free service, and my parents were just about the only GPs to vote in favour of the NHS in their district. Because of his kindness for many years during the Depression and my mother's compassionate approach, patients were queuing hundreds of yards on the approach road to the surgery to register with them as NHS patients in 1948.

The practice quickly built up to about 10,000 patients, and in the early 1950s they took on a partner, Dr. A. B. C. Smith, a Scotsman. (The population of the whole of Castleford at that time was less than 40,000.) The surgery had two consulting rooms, a waiting room and a room that contained all 10,000 records and where the receptionist, Miss Gray, worked. My father rarely wrote in the patient's records and the practice consistently spent too much money on prescription drugs. Men from London were sent up to assess the situation and he was threatened with fines. He told them that he would always prescribe the best for his patients. My mother had the same approach.

My parents fell out with Dr. Smith and eventually he was persuaded to leave if my father retired, which he did at the age of about 63. Dr. Smith was allocated all my father's patients (several thousands). Dr. Smith set up about 2 miles away and my mother took on a partner, Dr. Suniel Minocha. She had a shopping basket in the living room into which she put the hundreds of medical cards of those who changed from Dr. Smith to her each day. My father continued working with her as an unpaid honorary assistant. He did a few home visits.

The first Tieve Tara dog

My father and his first wife took over looking after his brother's dog, James, a bull mastiff. I am not sure what year that was.

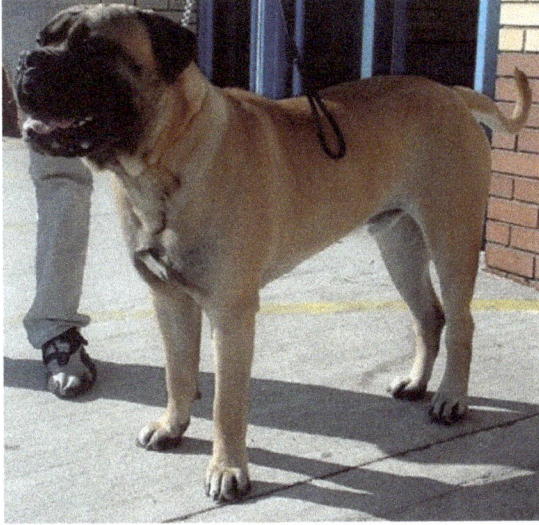

Bull mastiff

My father's brother, Sam, had James when he was a GP in the country town of Helperby in North Yorkshire. Uncle Sam moved to work as a GP in Wakefield, and the house (312 Dewsbury Road) was on a main road and not at all suitable for dogs.

The dogs my father knew after James were Wooffee and Regie (see above). Wooffee once got on to the dining room table and ate my father's lunch. He was furious. I saw him chasing the dog round the garden. My father had a rolled-up British Medical Journal in his hand ready to belt the dog. However, the dog ran off. My father visibly aged after he retired in about 1961. My mother made him go out for a daily walk with her and Regie. They did not walk far from the house. On their return my father would exclaim, "Twenty-four!" or another number. He had counted how many times the dog had urinated on the short walk.

* * *

My father had no active hobbies and had great difficulty sleeping. (This was a long-standing problem.) He used to take chloral hydrate to get to sleep, and this medication was in the form of crystals which he weighed on some old scales and then dissolved in water. He did read non-fiction and poetry. He could recite poetry. He would recite Kipling's "If" to me.

He died unexpectedly on 6 January 1967 aged 69. It was very cold on the day of his funeral. My mother did not go to the funeral as she was so distraught. As the cortège drove slowly up Fryston Road (the main road in Airedale, Castleford), the men who had worked in the mine came out of their houses, lined the road and doffed their flat caps as we passed. The headline of an article in the local paper was "Doctor who was dedicated to serving mankind".

Kathleen Mary Sloan née Sanders (1946–2015)

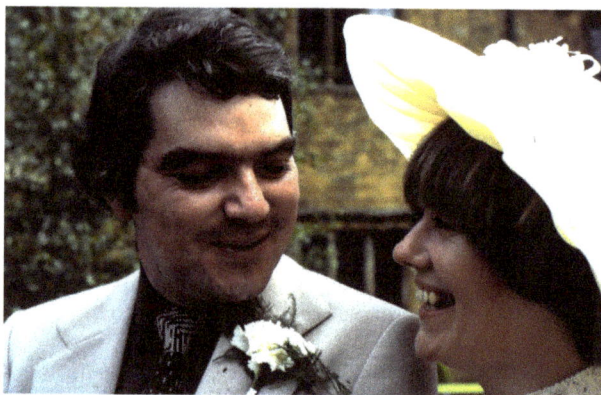

Wedding, June 3rd 1978

Kath was born in Rugby and was brought up by her parents, Hilda and Charlie Sanders, in a village called Woodford Halse in the county of Northamptonshire. My German-born mother always pronounced it "Vudelsford Halza". Woodford was a railway village. Charlie was a railway engine driver and Hilda a secretary. They were both Labour Party people and worked for their unions. Charlie's first wife died. They had a daughter called Mabel. One of Kath's best childhood friends was also called Kath and this friendship was kept up until her death. The two were friends since they were babies.

Kath was, like me, an only child, and her mother was very keen that she had a good education. Kath obtained a place in King's College London, to study Spanish, with Portuguese as a second language. King's is one of the best universities in the UK. Kath started at King's in 1964. I started at the rival, University College London, in 1963. We were introduced by a friend, Rosslynne Wheeldon. Rosslynne and I were in the same class in Airedale Infant's School and have remained friends to this day. Kath and Rosslynne were in the same Hall of Residence in London, Nutford House (The Nuthouse). Kath and I went out together and I fell in love with her. She was elected Lady Vice President of King's. She really enjoyed that as she had a big social role. I don't think she thought about Spanish much at that time. I asked her to marry me and she was quite right in refusing. We were too young. She ended our relationship.

After she obtained her degree, she was not sure what she wanted to do. She still did not know what she wanted to do when she got to her sixties. She started training as a surveyor with a firm called Gerald Eve and Co. She failed her examinations but loved working and socialising with those work colleagues. There was a lot of lunchtime drinking at the pub! In the evenings, she worked for a while as a barmaid at The Bull's Head in Barnes. This was frequented by many jazz players including Ronnie Scott, whom she met. She then worked at the Royal Institute of Chartered Surveyors for some years. There was a senior man working there called Ian Brown. He decided to set up his own small business, which was effectively an employment agency for surveyors. He asked Kath to join him. There were just the two of them and secretarial help in that business. Ian Brown was a great employer. My first, seven-year marriage to Felicity failed. I found out from Rosslynne that Kath was not married and, after significant imbibing of brandy, plucked up courage to phone her to ask her out. We went to Tiddydolls restaurant in Shepherd's Market,

Mayfair. I ordered quail's eggs for a starter. I had no idea how to eat them and ate the eggs shells and all. It was a lovely evening.

I told her I would not ask her to marry me again. She asked me to marry her at a party I held in my house in Cheltenham. I gave up my Cheltenham job and was offered a job as a lecturer in Physiology at The London Hospital Medical College. I was in that same job for three years in the early 1970s. However, I had made a big mistake. I resigned from the job and worked for a while in a practice in Roehampton. Gerda and Henry Tintner were partners there. Gerda was a close friend of my mother. She and my mother had been fellow medical students at Berlin University. Kath and I rented a flat round the corner from the practice. Marussia was the owner of the flat and was a school friend of my mother and Gerda. Marussia was a solicitor and had represented me in my divorce. She was fun and eccentric. Her house was called Poopiloo and she called her budgerigar by the same name. She was distraught when the bird died and maintained it was from lead poisoning from her windows.

It was 1978. My mother had retired and there was an empty house and GP surgery (Tieve Tara), which she was unable to sell. On a whim, Kath and I decided to move out of London and set up a general practice from scratch in Airedale where I was brought up. What an amazing support Kath was to me then and throughout our marriage. She was prepared to leave her very good job in London for this adventure. She was the practice manager for two or more years and the whole business of setting up was a great stress for us both. As mentioned earlier, we owned a flat in Budleigh Salterton in Devon, the sale of which gave us financial support. My mother moved from Cheltenham to a bungalow in Airedale. When the practice was established, Kath set up a small catering business and prepared and delivered buffets. This was very hard work, but it resulted in some beautifully produced food.

In about 1981 Kath decided she would like to work at our local stately home, Nostell Priory. The owner at that time was the fourth Baron St Oswald, Rowland Winn. He was a Conservative politician and had been a minister in Harold Macmillan's government. Kath wrote him a letter and I drove there one evening to deliver it. When

I got to the front door, there was no letter box, so I rang the bell. Someone answered and asked if I would like to come in and give the letter to his Lordship. I did not! I was dressed rather scruffily. Kath received a letter back from him telling her that there were no paid jobs, but he had an idea about some voluntary work. He invited her to dinner to discuss this. She drove over and just after I had finished my evening surgery phoned me to say that her car had broken down and that I was also invited for dinner. I could then bring her home. I rapidly spruced myself up and changed into a suit. The dinner was in the state dining room and the other guests were seriously posh. One was a general who managed the whole of the transport system of the British Army. The joke was that he was unable to fix Kath's car, but his wife might be able to. She had done a car maintenance course. I was sitting next to a duchess. Lord St Oswald suggested that Kath should be one of the founder members of the Friends of Nostell Priory.

After Kath had been working with the Friends for about a year, Lord St Oswald offered her a job as deputy manager of Nostell Priory Enterprises. This was a company that ran the events, weddings, dinners and meetings of bodies such as the Yorkshire Society. She worked so terribly hard in that job that sometimes we had to have Sunday lunch together in the café at Nostell. There were lots of evening events. One huge event she organised was the country fair, which was an annual event.

She met some fascinating people in that job. Kenneth Williams made a phone call from her office. She had a lovely chat with Lord Hailsham. I was really proud of her in that job. I am proud of her now.

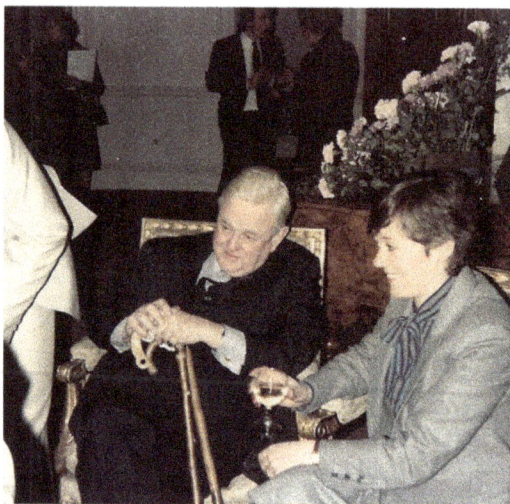

Kath and Lord Hailsham

Lord St Oswald died in December 1984. Kath could not work with anyone else and she resigned from her job.

She then became Tieve Tara's general practice manager once again. The practice had grown. She was a brilliant manager of both people and the business. She facilitated our achieving the King's Fund Organisational Audit and also our obtaining the Investors in People award. Kath also managed the building of two extensions to the surgery. Her main strength was people management. I am sure it was she who introduced and maintained a culture of friendliness between everyone in the team. This culture continues now and is evidenced in the chapter on partners and staff which I have called "Colleagues". The administration of a general practice is sometimes a great burden. Kath retired in 2000.

More Tieve Tara dogs

This is an appropriate point to write about our dogs. It is appropriate because Kath's retirement present from the colleagues at the surgery was a Labrador dog which we called Ben. She retired on the last day of December 2000. The present was a total surprise to her as we had decided a couple of years before not to have any more dogs after our second dog, Sam, died. I spent about six months assessing whether deep in her heart she would really like another dog. It would have been awful if I had got that wrong.

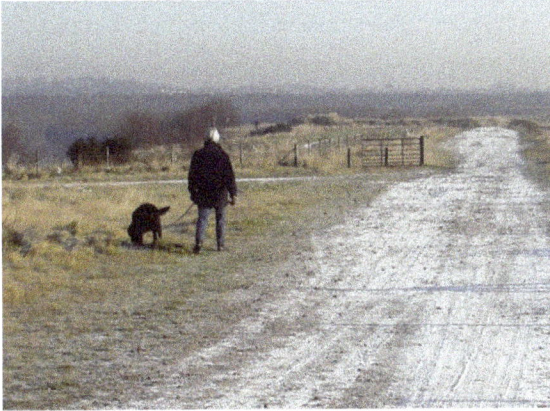

Kath taking Ben for a walk by the River Aire

The first dog we had was a golden Labrador which we called Sindy.

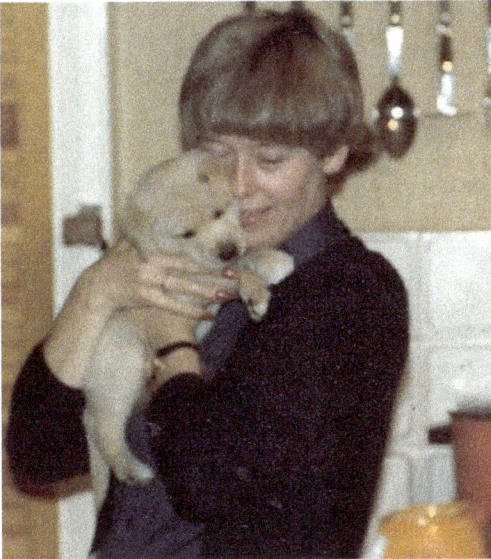

Sindy and Kath

Sindy grew up to be a lovely dog. She occasionally slept between us on our bed. I never slept a wink because she snored! I was on family planning duty one weekend. Sindy was in heat. I let her out of the kitchen door and was sipping a cup of coffee when I realised there were goings-on in the garden. Bruce had got into the garden and this resulted in five puppies in due course. (Bruce was owned by the Hayward family who lived not far away). We kept the largest black puppy and called him Sam. We gave the others away to friends. When Sam was one year old, we held a dogs' birthday party in our garden. Sindy's offspring were not at all interested in their mother. They only wanted to run about and sniff one another's nether regions. Bruce was not invited. He was a canis non grata.

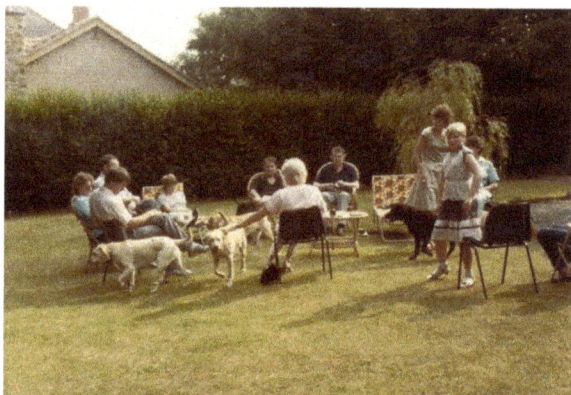

The dogs' first birthday party

* * *

After her retirement Kath undertook serious courses. One was on renaissance art at Leeds University. She undertook two courses in wine knowledge (not tasting). These courses involved examinations and coursework. She obtained distinctions in them all. We bought two wine fridges, one for red and the other for white. Kath built up a really good collection of fine wines. Her knowledge of art taught me a lot and enriched our many visits to Italy.

Kath became a Catholic in 2006. She worked as a volunteer for CAFOD (the Catholic Agency for Overseas Development) in the Leeds office at Hinsley Hall. The manager, Margaret, was a saint of a person and Kath loved working with her. Kath was a very popular secretary of the Castleford Choral Society for many, many years and took the society from strength to strength. She worked as a volunteer for the Citizens Advice Bureau in Pontefract and eventually became its chair.

She had the idea of our buying a second house in Gunnerside, Swaledale, North Yorkshire. We had that house for nearly twenty years.

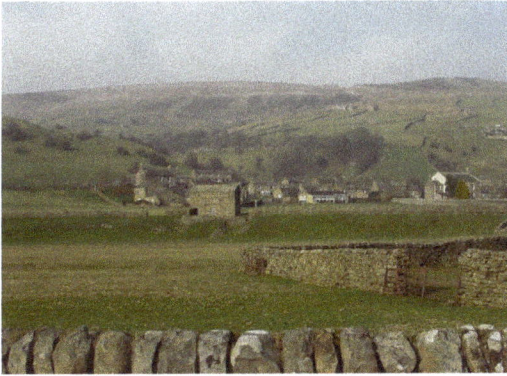

Gunnerside Village, Swaledale, North Yorkshire

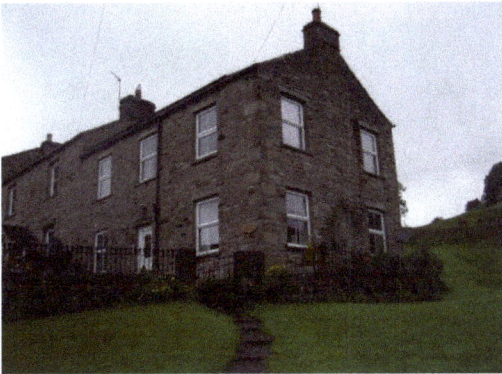

South View, Gunnerside

In 2006, Kath had the idea of selling that house and buying one in Umbria, Italy. Oh, what happy times we had in these places both on our own and with friends.

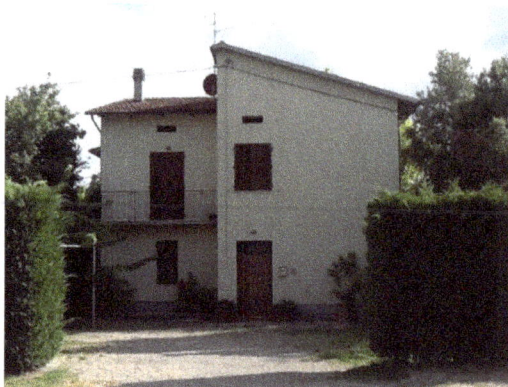

The house in Macchie, Italy. Purchased 2006

Macchie is very close to Lake Trasimeno. I took some of Kath's ashes to Italy, and I and our close friends, Kath and Alan, scattered them onto the lake from the end of the pier at Borghetto. In the last years when I have visited Italy with Kath and Alan (and relations of Kath, Martin and Jen), we always visit the pier and scatter some flowers into the lake.

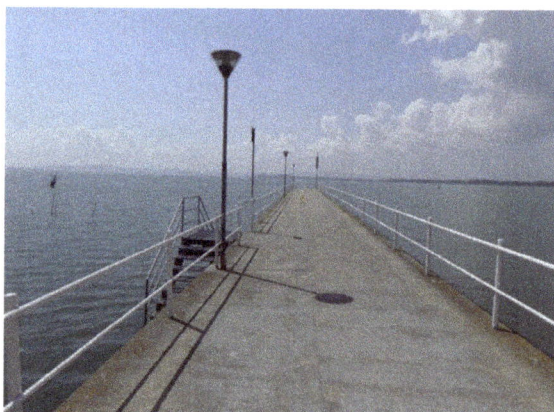

The pier at Borghetto

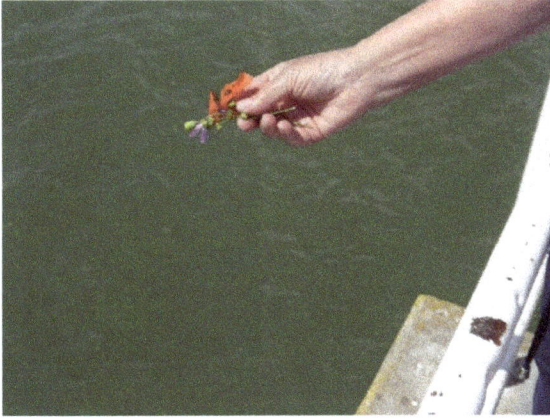

Poppies for Lake Trasimeno

After Kath's untimely death I self-published a book which was a tribute to her. I have only given that book to about twelve people. In it were the contents of the many letters and cards I was sent and my brief explanation of whom they were from. I wrote a short piece on "Love and Grief" at the end.

Here is a poem from that tribute book.

> Do not stand at my grave and weep.
> I am not there I do not sleep.
> I am a thousand winds that blow.
> I am the diamond glints on snow.
> I am the sunlight on ripened grain.
> I am the gentle autumn rain.
> When you awaken in the morning's hush
> I am the swift uplifting rush
> Of quiet birds in circled flight.
> I am the soft stars that shine at night.
> Do not stand by my grave and cry.
> I am not there I did not die.
> —Mary Elizabeth Frye

Richard Ernest George Sloan (1945–)

On 1 November 1978 I saw my first patient in Tieve Tara Surgery after Kath and I had set it up again. He wandered in at 9.25 am. I gave him a very thorough assessment as I wanted it to get round how good we were. I think he only had a cold!

We were not popular with the local doctors as the main way to build up the practice was for patients to change from the practice where they were registered. The Castleford doctors stopped my using their out-of-hours deputising service and I did two and a half months on call with no time off.

My first pay was at the end of December after I had been working like that for two months. It was for £2.96 less 6 per cent superannuation contribution. Pay was calculated quarterly and was partly related to the number of registered patients. 1 October was the first day of the quarter when I started. I started on November 1st. So the number of patients I had on 1 October was zero. The £2.96 was for a smear test I had undertaken. The accounts for the first year showed a loss of £3048.21. I would have had to resign if I made a loss in the second year. Fortunately, this did not happen. We were under great stress and would not recommend this sort of thing to any doctor.

I became a trainer, Continuing Medical Education tutor for GPs, a course organiser and an associate director of postgraduate GP education. GP education was the love of my life. I became the GP education advisor and appraisal lead for our Primary Care Trust.

The practice put on a great retirement party for me. As I am half German, an oompah band was employed for the party.

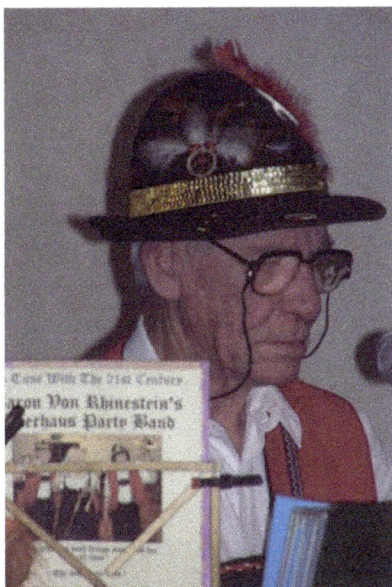

Baron von Rhinestein

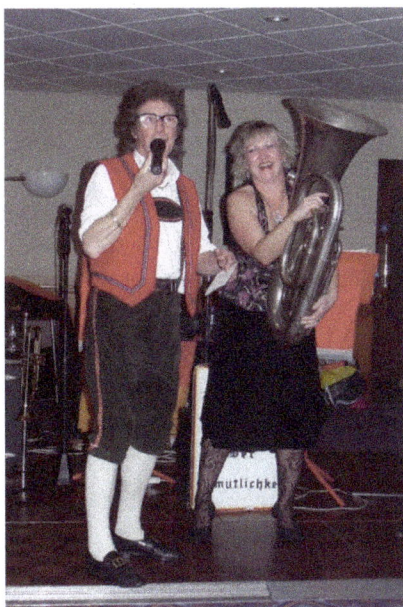

Samantha having a go with a euphonium

I often am asked what I do in my retirement. I retired as a GP in 2005 and continued working part time for the Primary Care Trust as an education advisor, fully retiring in 2010. I have immersed myself in voluntary unpaid work since then. The organisations I am involved in have the aim of helping vulnerable people and those without a voice.

I am vice chair of a community group called the Airedale Neighbourhood Management Board and chair its health subcommittee. We have been in existence for well over a decade. We have been involved with all sorts of community projects, and the theme of the health subgroup at this time is helping combat loneliness and social isolation. I am involved in promoting our library and I am a member of a multi-academy trust.

I am a trustee of a small charity, Spectrum People, which helps very vulnerable people. My main involvement is with Healthwatch Wakefield Ltd, a charity that is the voice of the people regarding the NHS and social care providers. I am a trustee. I am also a trustee of Age UK Wakefield. I am the patrons' secretary of the Castleford Choral Society, of which I have been a member since about 1981.

In 2016 I became a Catholic. My late wife became a Catholic in 2006. This has been a most significant thing in my life in recent years. I do some visiting of the elderly and lonely for the St. Vincent de Paul group of my church. My main hobbies are music, writing and travel. I am so lucky to have so many good friends both locally and all over the country. I have been on holidays with some of them. I am happy travelling alone now. In 2018 I went to Australia for two weeks and visited my only cousin, Angela, and her family in Brisbane. While in Australia, I also visited Sydney and the Great Barrier Reef. I live in Hill House and have no intention of moving.

* * *

I have never written about the following experience:

Early in 2011 I went to get our post from the box at the front gate. As I walked back to the house, I skimmed through the envelopes and amongst them was an official looking one. I opened it in the kitchen. It was from the office of the Prime Minister (David Cameron) stating that I had been awarded an MBE for services to healthcare in West Yorkshire. I was absolutely shocked and excited. Kath was upstairs in her office and I ran up to show her. She was thrilled for me. I had to send back a form to say I would accept the honour. I was known in the Airedale post office, so I drove to Wakefield and posted it special delivery. Of course, I had to keep this secret and only Kath knew about it. It was to be announced in the Queen's Birthday Honours list in June that year, and after that, I could tell friends. The full title of the honour is Member of the Most Excellent Order of the British Empire. There is a British Empire Medal below that, and higher orders are the OBE (Officer), CBE (Commander) and KBE and DBE (Knight and Dame).

In that June of 2011, Kath and I were on holiday in Italy in our house with our closest friends, Kath and Alan Overton. I got up at the crack of dawn on the announcement day to look for my name in the London Gazette (on the internet), where the honours are officially published. There it was. We had decided that Kath would tell our friends. Kath shed a tear as she was telling them. Kath and I had decided that Kath and Alan would be our guests at the investiture in Buckingham Palace, and they were thrilled. That day, the Pontefract and Castleford Express phoned me for an interview. It was on Radio Aire and was put in the Yorkshire Post. I received scores of cards, letters and emails from friends and colleagues when we got back to the UK. There were letters from the Secretary of State for Health (Andrew Lansley), the President of the Royal Society of Medicine, the President of the Royal College of General Practitioners, my MP, Yvette Cooper, and the leader of Wakefield Council, my friend, Peter Box CBE. I found out that I had been nominated twice. Once by the Patient Participation Group of Tieve Tara Surgery in about 2005 and again by people associated with my work at the Primary Care Trust and the Yorkshire Deanery. This nomination from the PCT was led by Tony Nicholas, the events manager, with whom I worked closely.

The investiture took place in December 2011. We four stayed in a hotel in Kensington. The Royal College of General Practitioners had supplied a limousine and driver for the event. I wore morning suit and my wife, Kath and Alan were stunning. We were dropped off at Buckingham Palace and one was not told who was undertaking the investiture in advance. We hoped it might be the Queen when we saw Royal Ensign flag flying over the palace. The art and décor inside the palace were simply fabulous. The Gentleman's Lavatory was pretty stunning also!

I split from my guests and waited in a beautiful anteroom for the event to start. We were given instructions as to what was to occur, how to bow, etc. We were told that it was to be Her Majesty the Queen doing the investiture. When it was my turn for the Queen to pin the medal on me, I got seriously nervous. However, I was amazed how nice, friendly and well informed she was. The last thing she said to me was "Yes, I think general practitioners are very important." I met my guests and then we had the official photographs taken outside the palace. We went to a concert at the Barbican in the evening.

The next day I had arranged for us to go to Prime Minister's Questions in the House of Commons and we were shown round briefly by the secretary of my MP, Yvette Cooper. Afterwards, Yvette met us and took us out onto the terrace.

The MBE award was second only to my marriage to Kath as one of the happiest moments of my life.

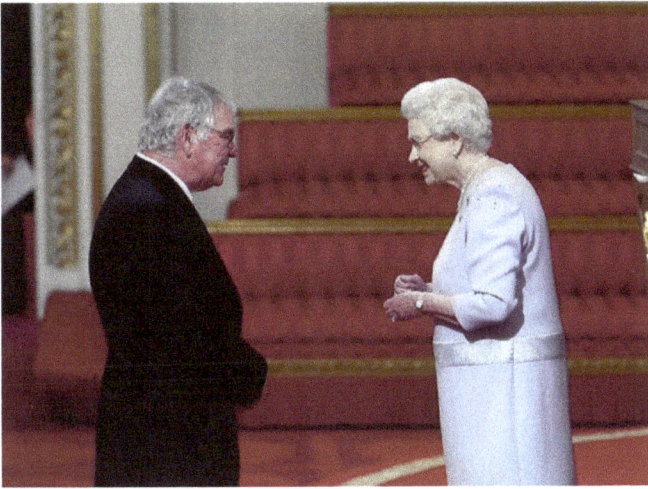

Me with another wonderful woman

If I had not had the amazing support of my medical practice, especially Anne Godridge, in allowing me to take time out, I would not have been nominated for this award. Kath was a towering support during our life together.

Chapter 3 – Cleaners and Housekeepers

In the early days, the housekeeper cleaned the house and also the small surgery. Later the cleaning of the surgery was done by person(s) separate from the housekeeper of the private house. They were referred to as surgery cleaners. This essay gives a picture of the middle-class lifestyle of GPs from before the launch of the NHS. It also shows the close relationships that developed between my family and our housekeepers.

The housekeeper for about the first ten years of my childhood was Hannah McGrath (Magash). The McGrath family had a really close relationship with our family. When my father was going through a marriage breakdown and divorce, the children sometimes had to be looked after by and stay with the McGrath family, who lived just round the corner. Mrs. McGrath went to the court in London to give evidence in favour of my father for the divorce case. She was a Roman Catholic and was excommunicated by the Church for this loyal act. When I was quite small, Magash came on holiday to Belgium with us to look after me while my parents went out (my mother to the casinos in Ostend!!). Magash came every weekday and cooked lunch. Sometimes my mother had prepared the lunch earlier. One of Magash's daughters, Maureen, was a cleaner and cleaned the surgery as well as other houses. More about Maureen later. Her other daughter, Kathleen (Paddy), took messages for my parents at her house, which was about one and a half miles away. Maureen's husband, Bert, washed the cars each. Magash's third child, Harry, was a prisoner of war and contracted TB there. Harry sometimes drove my father on his visits. I think this was occupational therapy for Harry as he was too ill with chest symptoms to hold down a job. Magash's husband, Jimmy, was fun and used to swap pornographic books with my mother! She used to wrap them in brown paper. These were easy for me to find amongst her large number of books!

Hannah and Jimmy often went up to stay in Glasgow with my half-sister, Geraldine, and her family. They and Maureen were invited to weddings of Geraldine's children. Mr. and Mrs. McGrath came to my first marriage.

Magash was a really skilled at icing cakes. She iced some fantastic wedding cakes that she made. My mother always took the Christmas cake she had baked to Magash for icing. However, my mother was not particularly good at baking cakes. She once took one round to Magash to be iced that was rock hard and inedible. Magash cooked another cake, iced it and took it to our house. My mother thought she herself had cooked a fantastic cake that year. Magash was one of the first people to join our practice in 1978. I looked after her in her terminal illness a year or so later.

Joan Harris was the surgery cleaner some years after the Second World War. Mary Tate cleaned the house and surgery later. Both became patients of mine in 1978 and both had lovely families. Joan told me that she used to clean up after my father had done a minor surgery session on a Sunday morning. He always gave her a packet of cigarettes as well as her wages.

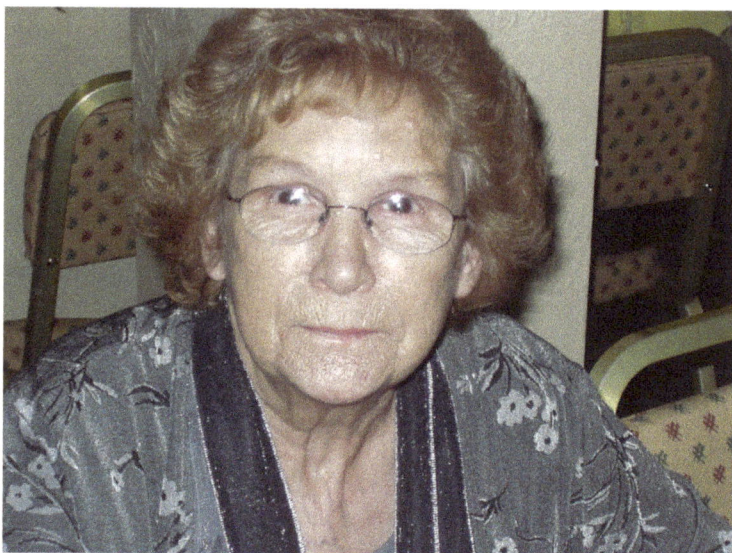

Mary Tate

Mrs. Edgington was the housekeeper after Magash and then there was Pru. Pru wore an onion as a pendant to ward off some disease or other.

Before I left home for university, Mrs. Drucilla Mitchell became the housekeeper. To my horror, her job before this was as a dinner lady in a local school. As I mentioned above, housekeepers cooked lunch, and I called her specialty "rotten stew". Actually, it was quite nice. Mrs. Mitchell continued as my mother's housekeeper well after my father died in 1967. She stayed with my mother in her house near Cheltenham. She once kindly made me a cup of coffee. (I was a GP there in the mid-1970s and my mother had bought a bungalow in Bishop's Cleeve.) She accidentally put two spoons of Ariel washing powder into my cup instead of sugar. My mother kept the Ariel in a small open glass bowl in the kitchen. I phoned Guy's poison centre to check if I might have to have a stomach washout. Actually, I only had taken the very smallest of sips and was just winding them up.

My wife, Kath, and I set up Tieve Tara Surgery from scratch in 1978. Maureen and Paddy (Mrs. McGrath's daughters mentioned above) were the most fantastic help. Paddy's husband, Ernest, was a joiner by trade. He did or managed loads of work on the house and surgery before and after we moved in. When we were still living and working in London, that family dealt with the alterations, decorating, etc. We communicated by phone and trusted them to do everything right. Paddy and Maureen helped us move in. Paddy never let me forget one particular incident. She and her sister were struggling up the stairs with a heavy chest of drawers and I was following behind carrying a cushion! This actually is a true reflection of the approach I have had to physical work all my life, as my friends are aware.

When the surgery reopened, Maureen was the surgery cleaner and also our housekeeper but gave up the surgery work after we settled in. Ruby Caborn took over and was the surgery cleaner for many years. One morning, the first person in to work found Ruby lying on the floor. She had fallen off a stepladder and broken a bone in her leg. She retired due to illness a few years after that.

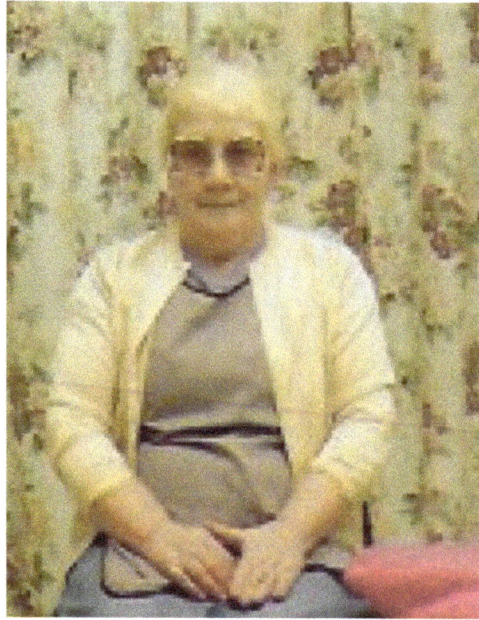

Ruby Caborn

Then came Madge Charlesworth. Madge had a personality and a half. You can read the press reports about her by googling her name. She led a campaign to win equal pay for women who worked for the National Coal Board. She was often on local television.

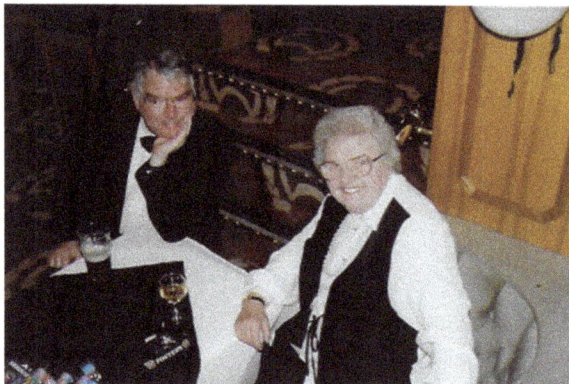

Madge Charlesworth and me

After I watched her on TV, I would phone her up to tell her how good she was. She was good. She told me once that she had been in London near the Houses of Parliament and she spotted David Dimbleby recording an interview. She went over to him and asked, "Are you David Dimbleby?". He said, "Do I know you?" Madge said, "No, but tha soon will," and proceeded to tell him at length about the campaign.

Madge started the evening cleaning session at 5.30 pm while we were still consulting. She would knock on my door and come straight in. It did not matter to her that there was a patient with me. She would say, "Can I 'av yer bin?" We actually asked her to stop doing that. The other habit she had was to meet and greet patients walking down to my consulting room after I had called their name out on the loudspeaker. She would stop the patient and say things like: "What are you doin' 'ere, Alf? You look allreet to me." I would have to get up and go out of my room to rescue the patient.

Madge's husband had some heart problems, and when we did the cardiopulmonary resuscitation training, we had never seen such violent chest compressions as when it was Madge's turn. She nearly broke the manikin. She really loved her husband and wanted to be able to help him if called for.

Madge was a fantastically loyal person and was an example to the whole team at Tieve Tara Medical Centre. The practice went in for the Investors in People award. This was a major task and involved everyone in the team including Madge. The assessor was known as Vicious Viv. Actually, she was very nice. On the day of our assessment, Madge was the first in to be interviewed. She entered the room and we heard her say in a loud voice, "Right!" When Viv gave us her feedback, she told us Madge was most impressive. We did achieve the award.

After Madge retired, Lil Fletcher was the surgery cleaner for a while.

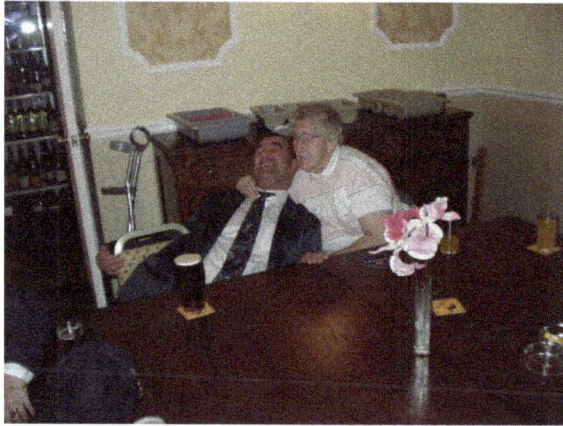

Lil Fletcher (with Tommy Kear) at a party

Lil's husband was Bill. He always wore a flat cap. I used to think he wore it in bed. He had a way of putting it on his head back to front and then rotating it into the correct position. One of their children, Andrew (Andy), was a really good professional rugby league player. He played for Wakefield Trinity and Yorkshire as well as other clubs later in his career.

When we moved into the last large extension, we contracted out the cleaning to a firm. The cleaners working for the firm thought they heard a ghost on a couple of occasions. This was after I retired. I think the senior partner, Anne Godridge, got in someone to exorcise the ghost.

Maureen Wood was our housekeeper from 1978 until about 2013 when she had to retire because of Alzheimer's. She was into her eighties when she retired. She came for a whole day twice a week, and her cleaning was immaculate. When we were on holiday, she continued coming and spring cleaned. She lived in the same house she was born in. The house was three minutes' walk from the surgery.

Maureen lived next door to Joan Davis, and they were childhood friends. Joan was born in 1925 and I met her in 2018. She told me then that when a car's headlight used to shine into their house, they knew it was my father's car. There were only two cars in Airedale at that time.

Maureen lived with her mother, Magash. My father delivered Maureen in that house. As I mentioned earlier, her house was round the corner from ours. Maureen's husband, Bert, died in his forties and they were not blessed with children. Magash had severe Alzheimer's disease towards the end of her life and Maureen and Paddy looked after her, helped by some NHS day-care sessions.

Maureen was more than our housekeeper. She was a dear friend. Kath, I and Maureen had lunch together in our kitchen on her workdays. She regarded us as her children. We were all members of the Castleford Choral Society from the early 1980s. She was always invited to the surgery Christmas party, and we went out for meals with her and took her on trips London. We went to Glasgow together for a wedding of one of my half nieces.

Maureen was a devout Catholic and went to church regularly. She had a great sense of humour and loved a laugh. I once found a telephone number one could use to get a daily message from Pope John Paul II. I dialled it for her during our lunch. She put the receiver to her ear and after a few seconds got to her knees on the kitchen floor. We laughed our heads off. She loved the birthday card Kath and I gave her one year. Inside was a pull-out image of Pope John Paul II. As the card was opened, his white cassock rose to reveal a pair of red bloomers.

In the Second World War, Maureen had a reserved occupation. That meant she could not be conscripted. Conscription for women was introduced in 1941. The reason was that her reserved occupation involved lighting the coal fires in the surgery waiting room and cleaning the surgery.

Maureen was a loyal patient of Tieve Tara Surgery/Medical Centre. She always asked, "Can I have all my tablets?" when she rang up for her repeat prescription. These included paracetamol, which were only prescribed to be used as required. Kath and I never had to buy any paracetamol as Maureen supplied her. (Many patients did this sort of thing. However, my knowledge that this was going on could have got me into trouble.) At one time, Kath developed a new medical problem that usually started with a headache. (She suffered from migraine.) Then she would fall into a deep sleep. I had trouble rousing her. When she woke up, she had slightly slurred speech and was a bit confused. I was really worried after one of these episodes and was in a panic when she set off somewhere in her car. I went out looking for her, thinking she might have fallen asleep driving. I could not find her, but she returned home and was OK. Another episode was when we were in Italy. It was in the afternoon in our house. I was worried enough to be looking up doctors' phone numbers. I decided that when we got home, she should see a neurologist. She came round and, as usual, was confused. We went out together to buy some flowers. We were in the shop a long time as Kath stopped and stared at the flowers for ages. She completely recovered. When we got home, she made the diagnosis herself. Maureen regularly took a sleeping tablet called Mogadon (nitrazepam). She had given Kath the sleeping tablets instead of the paracetamol. I was so relieved. I write this as a warning to people taking medication from friends.

In 2004 the huge extension and refurbishment of the older surgery was completed. We invited our MP, Yvette Cooper, and Maureen to open the new building jointly and unveil a plaque. I told our guests about Maureen's reserved occupation.

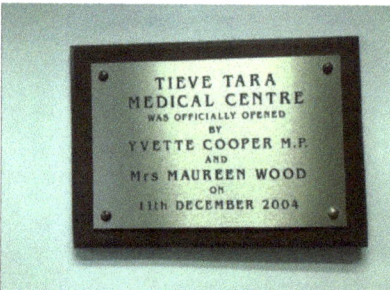

Opening Ceremony Plaque

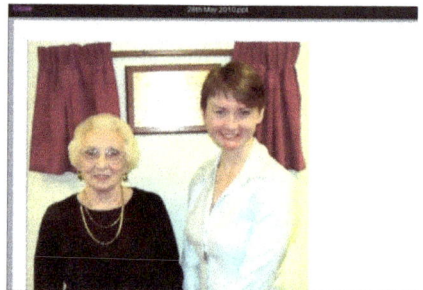

Maureen Wood and Yvette Cooper

Maureen developed a progressive Alzheimer's disease and moved out of the house in which she was born and lived with her niece Susan. Susan Oakley was a childhood friend of mine and she often came to our house to play. This is another example of the closeness of our two families. We kept Maureen on for quite a while, but she stopped communicating with us at lunchtime and just wanted to get on with the cleaning. She also started falling. We went to Susan's house to tell them she could not continue working for us. The only thing she said was "So you've given me the sack." She was eventually admitted to a nursing home. She died peacefully in 2014.

I can truly say that Kath and I loved Maureen and vice versa. About two years before her death, I noticed she carried a photograph of me in her purse. I sometimes shed a tear as I drive past her house or think about her. God rest her soul and the souls of all the cleaners and housekeepers mentioned.

Hill House is now cleaned by people from a firm called Merry Maids, and the two regular people who come, Tracey and Tracy, have been fantastic. They came to the cremation service for Kath. Since Kath died, they have done anything I have asked and give the house a really good clean once a fortnight. They even change my bed and make up beds if I have guests coming. Dawn Bell takes my shirts etc. to her home for ironing. She is the mother of Joe, who does the garden. Simon Bell, Joe's father, used to be the gardener until he changed jobs. It is good to have a family involved with the house again.

Chapter 4 – Colleagues

I have little information about the people who worked at the surgery in the first three decades of the existence of the practice. I think it was my father working alone and using locum doctors for holidays.

When I was a very young child, Miss Gray was the receptionist as well as everything else. She wore a white coat, as did my mother. (For work, my father always wore a three-piece suit.) His shirts had separate starched collars that were attached by collar studs. He used Brylcreem on his hair, and on his waistcoat there were invariably traces of cigarette ash. Despite the ash, he always looked smart.

Sylvia Ellerby was a receptionist in the late 1950s and possibly the early 1960s. She lives in the nearby pit village of Fryston. I last met her last at Altofts Methodist Church about fifteen years ago. I was giving a talk there. She had taken up playing the church organ.

In 1963 I left home to go to London to study medicine. I was nearly 18 years old. Joan Calvert was the receptionist/administrator at that time. I think she continued there until my mother retired in 1977. She became the practice manager in the McClintock practice based in Castleford. Kath and Joan got on well as fellow practice managers. We were so pleased that Joan invited us to her leaving dinner when she retired.

Gwyneth Brown was my mother's health visitor. After my mother retired, she was health visitor to the Minocha practice. The partners of that practice were Suniel Minocha (my mother's ex-partner) and his wife, Devika. Kath and I went to Italian lessons round about 2008. They took place in the Manygates Adult Education Centre in Wakefield. It was lovely to bump into Gwyneth there as she was doing a class on creative writing at the same time. We are Facebook friends and she is a lovely person, highly respected by her fellow health visitors.

Pauline Tinker was district nurse with my mother and, I think, before that with my parents. She certainly was the practice district nurse for many years. My mother and Pauline got on really well and became friends. Pauline and Donald's daughter, Pamela, also became friends with my mother. Donald was a senior council gardener. He became blind and lived into his nineties. He was a tough man and went out to the town centre on the bus. I occasionally saw him and gave him a lift. He died not so long ago.

* * *

The practice was started up again by me and my wife, Kath, on 1 November 1978. The chapters on family and housekeepers and cleaners describe the partners and staff from the early 1920s when my father started the practice and was joined by my mother as an assistant in 1943.

Soon after we started the practice, I desperately needed help at week ends and advertised widely including in the Wakefield Express. I received only one application to these adverts. It was written in pencil on lined paper torn out of a notebook. The address of the sender was "S. Royds Hospital". (Stanley Royd was a large psychiatric hospital in Wakefield.) The letter went on something like: "I see you are having trouble with your weak end. I can help you. I work in the morg here in the hospital so I know how to speak to the people." I wish I had kept that letter. It turned out to be from my Uncle Sam. He was my father's brother and was a GP in Wakefield until he retired to Northern Ireland. He read my advert in the Wakefield Express, which he had posted out to him each week.

Ann Martin, a junior doctor working very hard in Pontefract Hospital offered to help me out when she could. That was a fantastic thing to do. She eventually became a GP in Pontefract. Her husband, Ted McGrath, also occasionally helped. He too became a local GP. That was such a kind thing to do. Ann turned down my offer of a partnership a few years later. On reflection, I thought that was the right decision.

Kath and I managed to take a holiday occasionally by employing locums. I was amazed to discover that the system allowed a GP trainee to do locum work in a single-handed practice like mine. My friend and GP partner from Cheltenham, Robin Harrod, allowed his GP trainee to come and help me. The only condition was that my retired mother supervised him. I have my good friend Robin Harrod to thank for that holiday.

To try and have a better lifestyle, we started employing locums to work alongside me as well as for holidays. The practice was not large enough to employ a partner. The list size was growing slowly but surely.

Dai James was the GP partner who retired from the Cheltenham practice whose partnership place I took in 1973. He stayed with us for two weeks as an assistant/locum, working alongside me. He had a fantastic bedside manner and was a charmer. I know that from my working in Cheltenham and hearing about him. Dai and I were godfathers to Robin Harrod's daughter, Samantha, so I knew him slightly. Robin was at The London Hospital Medical College with me and was the best man at my first wedding. After Dai retired from the practice (he was in his forties), he and his wife Maggie bought and ran a dog kennel business. When the owners brought their precious dogs to him, he painstakingly noted their every dietary whim. "A little roast chicken and boiled rice. Stewed steak and mashed potatoes without salt." I think he gave all of the dogs Chum. I overheard him in our surgery reception area saying to a patient, "Madam. What is a person like you, the picture of health, doing at the doctor's on a lovely day like this?" He and I threw a surprise party one evening for Kath and got things ready while she was at a choir rehearsal. The staff were invited. I did a terrible thing at that party. I laced Joyce the secretary's drink with a spirit. She ended up crawling to the lavatory on her hands and knees. I have never laced anyone else's drink since then. It is a shocking thing to do. It was a hilarious sight, though!

John Papworth-Smith, who became the University of Leeds students' GP, was another marvellous doctor who helped as a long-term locum, working alongside me. One day I was in agony with an abscess in an embarrassing place and he incised it, with me lying on the couch in our lounge. Another kindness he showed us was when my mother was very ill. He took her to be admitted to Leeds General Infirmary while I continued with the work.

One Saturday morning I was cracking up. I was exhausted, depressed and in a state of anxiety. I was desperate for help, particularly at the weekends, so Kath and I could have a break. I was phoning round and eventually burst into tears on the phone talking to Jean Wharton, a consultant physician. She called my GP (John Waring) and he visited me. He made several phone calls trying to get someone to stand in for me but failed. He then did one of the most altruistic things I have ever experienced. He stood in for me himself and insisted I had some time off work. After that incident, his practice (Northgate Surgery in Pontefract, where my friend Grahame Smith worked) allowed me to be part of their out-of-hours rota. That was also fantastic.

My first medical partner in Airedale was my mother, who came out of retirement. She was a great help. I thought it ridiculous that the patients wanted to see me about measles and chickenpox when my mother was vastly more experienced than I with these infections. This was an example of ageism. One time, she went on a visit and, on leaving the patient's home, advised her to write to the council and ask for a handrail to be fitted to the side of the house where there was a path to the back door. The patient asked, "What for?" My mother, replied, "For me." My mother had some difficulty walking.

There was a clause in her partnership agreement that stated that after retirement she could not work in Castleford and its surrounds for five years. This was a standard clause for all GPs in those days. Early one evening there was a knock on the back door, and I was served with an injunction that closed the surgery down. The injunction was initiated by my mother's ex-medical partner, who had his practice based about a mile away. Patients were leaving that practice in significant numbers to join ours. There was a court case, and my mother was fined and had to pay costs. I was worried that the closure of the practice for three days would have a deleterious effect but actually it had the reverse. More patients changed GP to us than ever after that.

After about three years, the practice had grown such that I could consider taking on a partner. Kath became the practice manager once more. I advertised for a partner. It was a time when lots of doctors were looking for jobs, and there were about ninety applicants. What a contrast to the experience I described earlier. I interviewed about six of them. We had a dog, and the interviews were held in our house. The way each interviewee approached the dog was a major factor in my assessment of them! I told the applicants about the plans for a surgery extension. One applicant, who frightened me to an extent, looked at the plans and told me where we should site all the pot plants.

One of the ninety applicants was John Lee, who had qualified at Leeds and had been with me in the very early days. He came for two weeks as a medical student attachment. He was the only one of the ninety who knew how difficult the work was in Airedale. He was offered the job. He was a great partner. GP partnerships are like marriages and, like in the latter, John and I had our ups and downs. He was prudent with the practice finances, in contrast to me. Actually, I am being too polite here. Maureen, our housekeeper, used to say that when John opened his wallet, moths flew out.

It always amazed me that two male GPs, neither of whom had children, could have one of the largest paediatric practices in the area. Vaccination targets for children were introduced, and John felt we would never achieve these. I was determined we would, and he and I went out in the evenings doing house calls to perform vaccinations. We did achieve the targets.

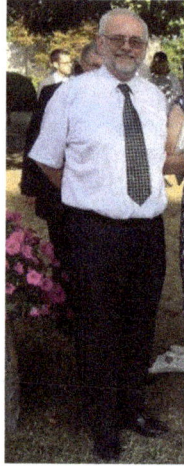

John Lee

I became a trainer. In another chapter I describe how much work had to be done by me and by the practice staff to become a training practice. Isobel McCormick was my very first trainee. I took over her training halfway through her GP training attachment when her trainer became ill. There is more about Isobel in the chapter on training.

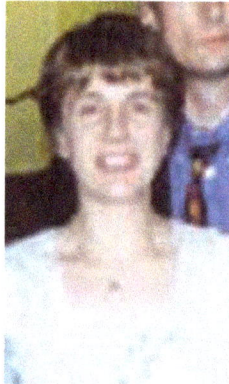

Isobel McCormick

My first *full-time* trainee was Anne Godridge. After six months with us, Anne moved on to complete her three-year training. She had about a year to go. After completing that year, Anne approached us to see if we needed another partner. We had not the numbers or income at that time to offer a full-time partnership. We offered her a share in the profits that increased over time until she had an equal share to ours. Anne has a great sense of humour. She once "accidentally" left out a fictitious positive pregnancy test result with her name as the patient. She just wanted to see the look on my face when I saw it. I knew that she would be a brilliant partner and she was.

My mother was not the only mother to help in the surgery. Anne's mother came in for a while to help with secretarial work. Anne now is the senior partner.

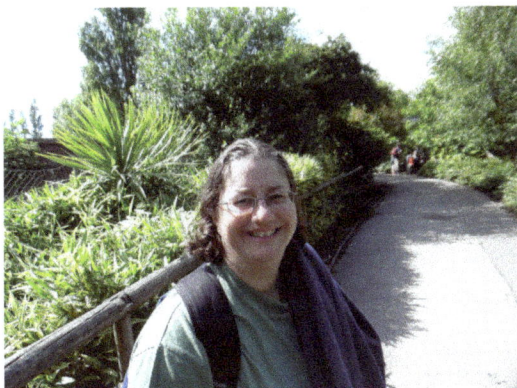

Anne Godridge

Anne, John, I and Kath made a great senior team. We had partners' meetings in our kitchen. The meetings started with a gin and tonic. This partnership, along with a fantastic group of attached and ancillary staff, achieved much. We obtained the King's Fund Organisational Audit award, the Investors in People award and a Beacon Practice award.

It was a very sad day when John retired from the practice and from general practice. This was the result of a totally unjustified complaint. However, he had a very successful career in Genito-Urinary Medicine and dermatology. He was the accompanist of the Castleford Choral Union for many years. He played the organ at my mother's funeral. His leaving was the end of another era for the practice.

John was replaced by Mohan Bazaz, who had been a surgeon for many years. He was a gentle man and a pleasure to work with but developed a neurological disease and had to give up medicine. He died not so many years ago.

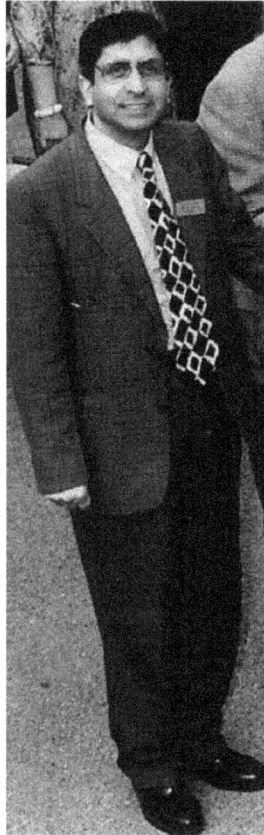

Mohan Bazaz

* * *

Before writing about the next phase of the practice, I want to go back and reflect on the practice team who were working during this "era".

There are two types of practice staff. Ancillary staff are directly employed and paid by the practice. Their sole place of work is the surgery. Seventy per cent of salaries were reimbursed by the NHS. (This did not apply to a relation of a partner, so Kath worked for nothing for several years until the rule was altered.) Ancillary staff include receptionists, the practice secretary, the practice manager, a practice nurse, a healthcare assistant, administrators, etc. Attached staff would be paid by other parts of the NHS and include district nurses, health visitors, midwives, etc.

The first directly employed secretary-cum-receptionist was Joyce Hunt. She was a shorthand typist and her previous employment was in the local secondary school. She used Kath's mother's old manual typewriter and was not at all keen on computers. Her husband, Ken, was a West Riding bus driver. Ken started work very early in the morning and delivered our patients' prescriptions to the chemists on his bus route. He regularly took our dog for a walk. Was Ken ancillary or attached? Neither. He was simply a good person and a friend of the surgery. We called him Uncle Ken and enjoyed the fabulous cakes he cooked and brought to us.

Joyce had a habit of handing her notice in for various reasons. Mainly due to me being an awkward devil. She was persuaded to stay until about the third episode when I accepted her resignation. I actually think she wanted to retire and enjoy her grandchildren. Several years later she came back to help tidy up the records and computerise summaries. We were amazed that she was willing to learn how to use a computer.

One day, when Joyce had well retired, my mother, who was getting somewhat muddled, phoned me very early in the morning to tell me that Ken had died. I was really upset and drove to their house. As I was walking up the path, Ken emerged from the house. I nearly passed out. It was my mother's neighbour who had died.

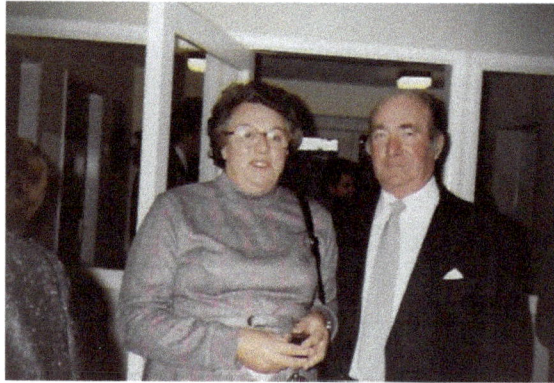

Joyce and Ken Hunt

Ann Long was the next receptionist to be employed by the surgery. She was amazingly loyal. She had a chronic intestinal problem which was serious enough for her to become ill occasionally and unable to work. She asked to do work at home when she was ill. She only worked for us for just over a year and then died tragically young from the intestinal disease before she reached the age of 40. I will never forget her. She was from the Maddison family who came from our pit village of Fryston.

Joyce and Ann knew many local people, and they were major factors for the list size increasing.

Andrea Woodward was Ann's replacement. Andrea had worked previously in Adam's fish and chip shop in Airedale. That was good enough for us. Again, she is one of the most loyal members of staff and she is the longest serving receptionist/administrator in the practice. Andrea started in 1983. She worked with Joyce, and their relationship was somewhat difficult at times. She deals with the repeat prescription requests now as well as undertaking reception duties. I have great memories of working so well with her. In the 1980s, the Christmas Eve open surgery was usually empty. I thought that anyone who turned up on the evening before Christmas must be seriously ill. Andrea and I usually had one small glass of sherry in the surgery that special evening. Or maybe it was just me. Andrea has now worked there longer than I did.

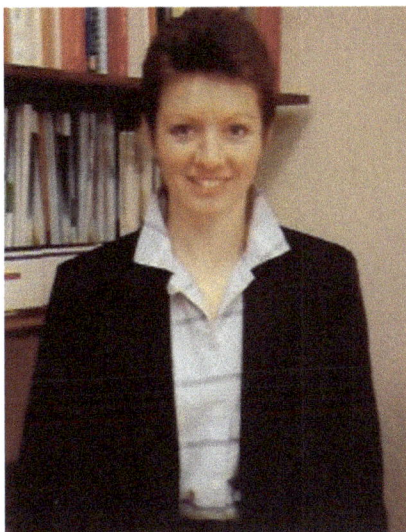

Andrea Woodward

The first attached health visitor was Sue Smith and she started in 1979. The practice somehow attracted a large number of children that were on the at-risk register for non-accidental injury. Sue was an expert in this area, and I learned a lot from her. She was a true friend to me and Kath for all those years and she remains one to me. She left the practice to undertake a BSc degree. The Pontefract area would not allow her to do this. How short sighted. She eventually obtained a PhD and runs a very successful training/facilitation business. She was recently awarded an honorary award from the Royal College of Surgeons in Ireland.

Sue was always hard up in the early days and undertook clothing sales parties in people's houses. She did one in ours. Just before she left the practice, she had a party in the waiting room for the attendees of the baby clinic. She brought the alcoholic refreshments and I brought the cigarettes! I think we both could have been struck off for doing that. Towards the end of the party, I noticed that some of the cigarettes had been stolen. I was certain I knew who it was and angrily drove to her house. Of course, I got nowhere with this. I forgot for a moment that this was Airedale, Castleford.

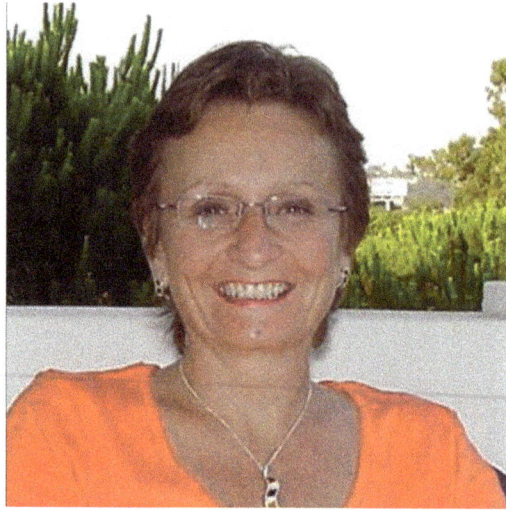

Sue Smith

Hazel Bird was employed as a receptionist in 1984. She was very good at her job and eventually did a lot more administration. She knew lots of the patients and, like the others in the front line, was a factor in new patients joining the list. The team had an annual Christmas party, but Kath and I also held the occasional practice party at our house. At one of the latter, people were asked to bring food and Hazel offered to bring a dip. The doorbell rang and there was Hazel, but the vessel holding the dip was at a jaunty angle as was she. She was slightly under the influence of the fermented grape. From that day on we have called it "dip a la slope". Hazel is and was larger than life, and Kath used to say that when there are two attention seekers in the same room there could be trouble. Kath thought the other attention seeker was I. What rubbish! Hazel left just before I retired, and she managed The Crown pub for a number of years. As I have mentioned, Hazel attracted a lot of new patients to the surgery and I am sure did the same for the pub.

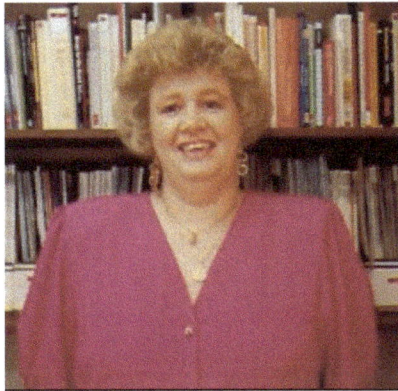

Hazel Bird

We had an assistant health visitor, Madeleine Davey, who looked after the adults. The practice had a very significant number of children who needed a full-time health visitor. I think Marjory Robinson took over from Sue. She was a very experienced nurse/ health visitor indeed. She was a matron at one point in her career. She told me that one could not judge or measure whether one was improving anything until seven years had passed. Sadly, she died prematurely from breast cancer complications.

Another amazing member of the attached staff was Anne Holt, the physiotherapist. I am convinced that she improved the patients' condition more than other physiotherapists. In my view, this was because of her holistic approach, consultation skills and her Christian religion.

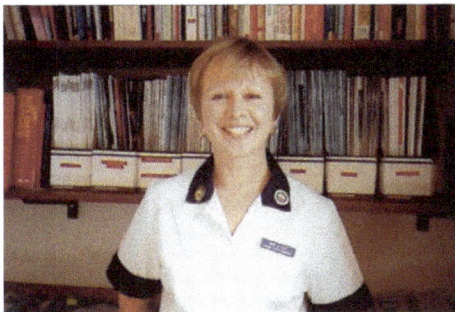

Anne Holt

Anne died suddenly and at the age of about 40 from a cerebral haemorrhage. She was a truly lovely and good person. I know her husband now. He is the chair of the trustee board of NOVA Wakefield District Ltd. He was also the chair of the interviewing committee for the job of Chair of Healthwatch Wakefield, for which I applied. I had not seen him for many years, and when I realised who he was, my heart sank. I remembered he and Anne had been to a number of the practice's boozy Christmas parties! On the evening of the interview, I was pacing up and down, waiting for him to contact me, and eventually the phone rang. It was Mike to tell me I had got the job. I told him about my worry about the parties. He said, "That was the sole reason you got the job." I occasionally meet him now, which is a great pleasure.

Marie Stephenson became our health visitor in 1984 and was with us for about nine years. We were so lucky to have such a competent person working with us. I am pleased that we have recently become Facebook friends so we can keep in touch.

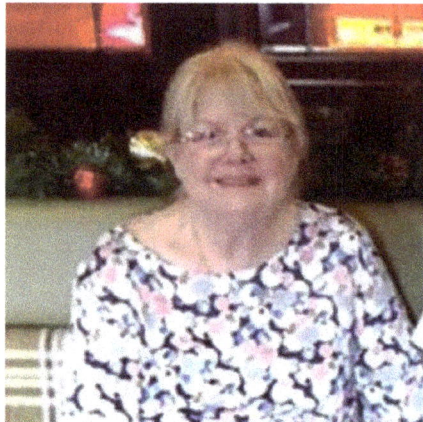

Marie Stephenson

We had two superb health visitors, Kathryn Padget and Julie Barron. That was in the latter part of the 1990s. They became good friends with one another and were a joy to work with. Again, like with Sue, I developed a great working relationship with Kathryn. Kath and I developed a friendship with Kathryn and her husband, Keith. We all went to London together on one occasion. Actually, Kathryn and I were attending a conference. Kath and Keith swanned off and enjoyed themselves! Kathryn was an ideas person and I think I was too. We were involved together in the organisational development of the Primary Care Group and we also involved the practice in a study of clinical supervision by Huddersfield University. Eventually Kathryn got a senior job in with Barnsley Primary Care Trust. I had a prolonged lunch with her not so long ago. She retired in 2018. When Kath was alive, we planned to have a surgery reunion of those from that era. I decided to have that anyway in 2016. Julie Barron and her husband came all the way from Cornwall.

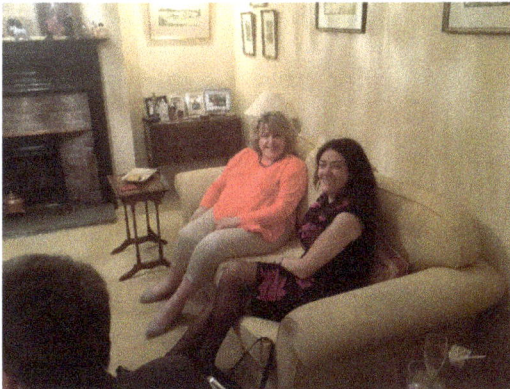

Julie (in the pink) and Kathryn. Reunion 2016.

Edna Box was the midwife for many years and worked closely with my mother. I have mentioned her briefly in the chapter on family. She did some of her training in Mile End Hospital in the East End of London. I was a medical houseman there in 1970, which was many years later. When she had her fourth child, Tim, he came to the house with her and my father babysat while Edna did the antenatal clinic with my mother. I played with Tim when I was not at school. Edna and my mother became firm friends and, after my father died, went on holiday together several times. (Edna had been a widow for many years.) Her son Tim told me recently that they had been to Italy together three times.

Edna was still working when I came to Castleford in 1978. In the early days of my general practice career, a woman could have her baby delivered under one of three different systems of care. The first two were a home delivery or a delivery in a maternity unit looked after by hospital staff. The third arrangement was called a GP unit delivery. That meant the GP was in overall charge of the delivery, which took place in the hospital maternity unit. I had delivered about forty babies during my training to be able to undertake maternity work in general practice. However, I was always a nervous wreck when managing a GP unit delivery. I was quite conscientious and would go to the maternity unit to see all was well. One time, Edna was the midwife delivering one of my GP unit mothers. When she saw me, she insisted I stay and watch her deliver the baby. It was a work of art and compassion. It brought tears to my eyes.

Edna died in July 2019. The funeral was amazing and packed with friends, colleagues and relations. The Box family is huge. Edna's mother-in-law, Emma, and her daughter-in-law, Jeanette, were midwives in Airedale.

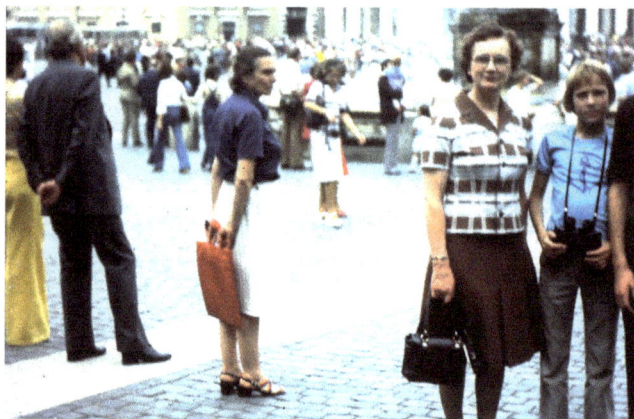

Edna Box on holiday with her son, Richard

GPs were paid extra for each pregnancy and postnatal care if they were on the obstetric list. The usual way to get on the list in the 1970s was to undertake a six-month obstetric hospital job.

This is a huge commitment. I took an alternative route to get onto the list. I undertook a six-month attachment with a consultant obstetrician in Barnet General Hospital ending with a two-week residential Senior House Officer locum. In those six months, I delivered twenty babies. I slept there one night a week. I did that while still working as a lecturer in Physiology. I had already delivered twenty when I was a student. Even then, the midwives were so much more skilled at the job than GPs.

The first midwife with the practice in 1978 was Sister Joyce Pearson. Because the practice started from scratch with no patients, eventually we had just one pregnant woman coming to the antenatal clinic. We held a clinic once a fortnight. On one occasion our only pregnant patient failed to attend. Sister Pearson and I had some great long chats in these easy clinics.

Two of the first patients to join the practice were Grahame and Caroline Smith. Grahame and I were both at University College London as medical students in 1963 and have remained close family and personal friends since then. Caroline was a nurse at The London Hospital, where I did my clinical medical training. Grahame and Caroline met when we were all in London. Shortly after joining the practice they gave me a great shock. Caroline was pregnant and wanted a home delivery. I was not keen on home deliveries. As her delivery approached, I went into the local hospital to check out the equipment. I was really anxious and praying that all would be well. First thing one morning my anxiety abated when I was told that Sister Pearson had delivered a healthy girl and that all was normal and OK. She was called Amy. Phew!

Mary Thornton became the practice midwife and she worked there for many years until she retired. Some of the best midwives are Irish, and I love her Irish accent. It reminds me of my father's accent. Mary was and is a wonderful person. I see her occasionally at the Catholic church in Knottingley. She is in her eighties, phones me occasionally and is a Facebook friend. She is a great-grand-mother. The other midwife at that time was Margaret Helliwell. Mary and Margaret made a great midwife team.

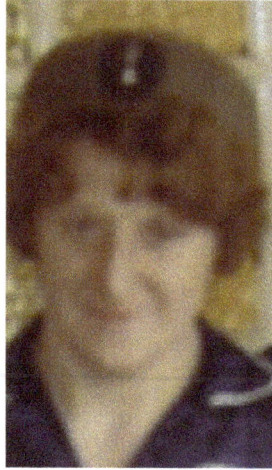

Margaret Helliwell

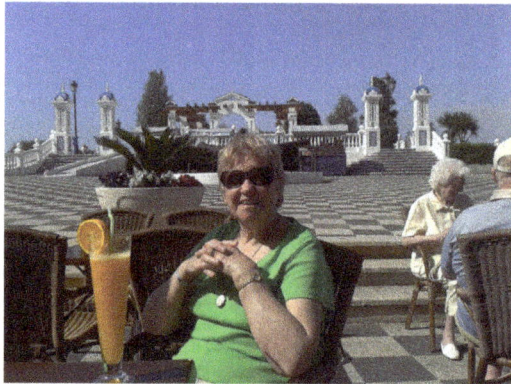

Mary Thornton

After Mary came Christine Rutherford. (She joined us in June 1998.) Another star of a midwife. She worked at Tieve Tara for over twenty years. She retired at the end of August 2019. She looked after the pregnant grandchildren of women whose babies we had delivered in the past. We once had a mother and daughter, both pregnant, coming together to the antenatal clinic. Gradually, GPs became deskilled in obstetrics as the midwives took over antenatal and postnatal care as well as deliveries. In the early days, the GP undertook an examination of the mother after the midwife had seen and examined her. Up to my retirement there was always a GP sharing the antenatal/postnatal surgery, but there was very little for the GP to do. I used to wander in and say to Christine, "You can relax now. I have arrived." During the clinic, I sat in my room catching up with paperwork and writing out the occasional prescription for indigestion medicine.

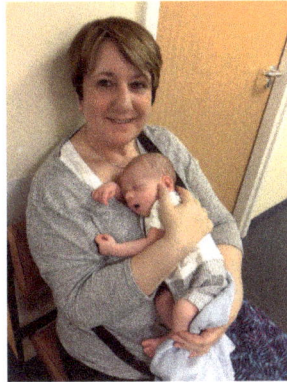

Christine Rutherford and her grandson, Thomas

Jeanette Box worked as a midwife with us from 1985 to 1988. She and all the midwives that worked at the practice were fabulous. Like several of the Box family, she was a patient of the practice. I last met Jeanette at Edna's funeral in August 2019.

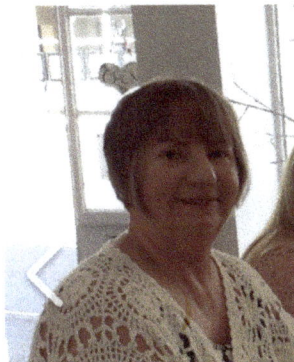

Jeanette Box

After Joyce retired as practice secretary, she was replaced by Jean Stones. Occasionally, I dictated a fictitious letter to her. One had a very slow start and was a referral to a psychiatrist. The symptoms and signs were bizarre and only towards the end of the letter did Jean realise I was writing about her. John Lee and I undertook attendance and mobility allowance medicals as an extra job. John often dictated his report while he was in his car with much traffic noise and opera music. Jean once did a tape like that for him to have a go at.

The partnership was persuaded by John Lee to not agree to the staff's request for new uniforms. We always had, as well as a Christmas party in a hotel, what we called the Practice Fuddle. This was held at the surgery and we each brought in food contributions. The partnership paid for the liquid refreshment. Jean and another couple of members of the staff pinned John into a corner under a bright light. They tried and failed to get him to change his mind about the uniforms. Jean got out a pair of scissors and cut his tie in half!

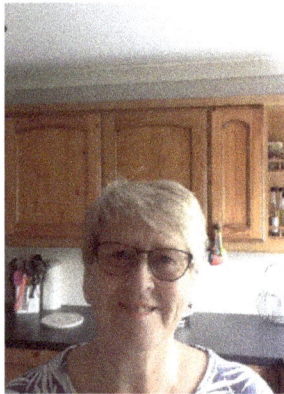

Jean Stones

Actually, he was really upset about that. Uniforms were eventually provided after quite a time had elapsed. Jean and Stephen, her husband, are friends of mine. They have been on holiday with Anne Godridge and her husband, Alan. Jean and Steve also made a close friendship with one of the trainees,

Norman Dawes. Norman emigrated to New Zealand. I have met him on a couple of occasions when he has visited the UK, usually at a pub for a meal with Jean and Steve.

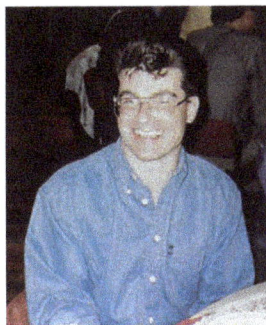

Norman Dawes

In 1991, Jean retired and Janet Pease was appointed as practice secretary. It is probably very bad of me, but the first things I think of associated with Janet are the really funny birthday and Christmas cards she has sent over the years. She still sends me them and I retired in 2005. Janet, like Jean, was super-efficient and loyal. I cannot remember whether it was she or Jean who once ended a letter with "Signed but not dictated by Dr. R. Sloan". I bet each will deny doing this! Janet undertook an increasing amount of work as general practice evolved with two major re-organisations of the NHS. GP training also generated significant secretarial work.

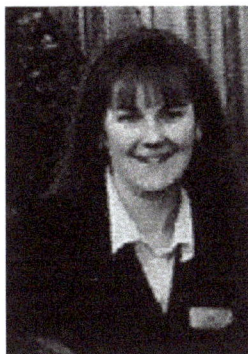

Janet Pease

The appointment of staff has not always been straightforward. The partners and practice manager once interviewed applicants and appointed someone as a receptionist who was not at all good. We had to ask her to leave in the end. Then we panicked because we had turned down someone who was potentially excellent. I was asked to phone her. Thank goodness Jean Howarth had not taken up a job. Jean joined the practice in 1996. She was indeed an excellent receptionist. She became an administrator in the practice and retired in 2019. I meet her and her husband as well as other retired and working staff at least once a year. We have a curry and a few drinks together and have been doing this for a number of years. Arnie Nicholson organises these meetings.

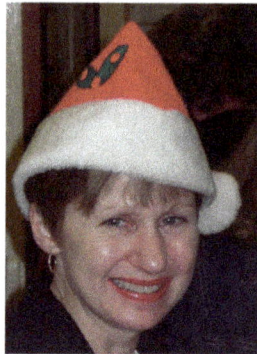

Jean Howarth

Arnie is the husband of a retired receptionist, Irene. Irene had really excellent communication skills working at the sharp end. She always seems so calm and reassuring. It is great that Kath and I, and now I, maintained a friendship with her and Arnie. They spend most of their time travelling the world. They had a terrible experience on a safari in Kenya many years ago. It was a tented safari, and one night their guides disappeared. I think they simply went home. They were stranded with the other travellers in the jungle. They were attacked by a gang who threatened to cut off fingers if their rings were not removed. Somehow someone went off and got help and all was OK. It took months for Irene to get over this, and I am sure Arnie was the same.

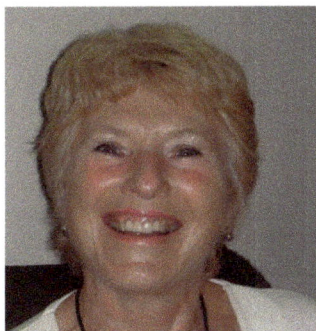

Irene Nicholson

Another receptionist who is now long retired is Brenda Booth. She was there at the same time as Jean Stones. Brenda and her husband, Ron, and Jean and Steve became firm friends. They have holidayed together, and I meet them occasionally for a pub meal. Ron is a Facebook friend of mine and has an interesting psychiatric problem. That problem is that he is totally obsessed with Castleford Tigers rugby team and club! This is not a rare condition, actually.

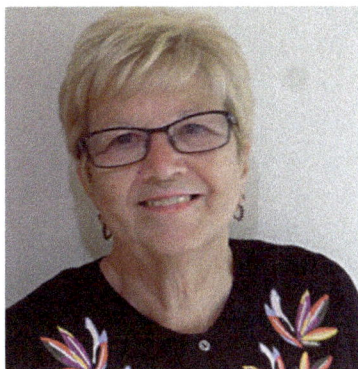

Brenda Booth

At first, Carolyn Cranton worked for both us and a neighbouring practice (Dr. Dunphy & Partners). She was the administrator whose work resulted in us attaining the King's Fund Organisational Audit award in the 1990s. We were eventually the sole employer of Carolyn, and she undertook a variety of administrative work for a number of years. She is a Facebook friend of mine and is a member of the gang that goes out for curry evenings.

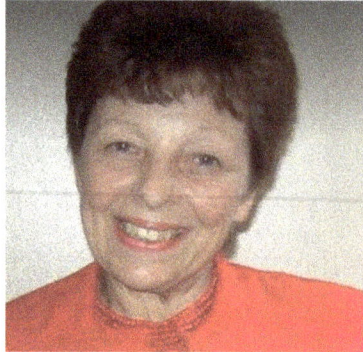

Carolyn Cranton

I have to pause here in case any reader has not realised something extraordinary about these people I have described so far and the ones that follow below. This was the most amazing team I have ever come across in any organisation. We laughed together. We socialised together. We worried together. We partied together. We looked after one another. We still meet together fourteen years after my retirement. Airedale was and still is a deprived area. Many, but certainly not all, of the patients had complex problems related to deprivation. We had a significant number of cases of child and domestic abuse, criminals, drug misusers, alcoholics, psychiatric problems, non-attenders, etc. It was stressful dealing with some of them, both at reception and in the consulting room. We had the greatest number of drug misusers of any practice in the area. We had the greatest number of safeguarding children (then called non-accidental injury) cases in the district in the early days. It was very difficult to reach targets for smear uptakes and vaccinations. It was the strength of the team that made this training practice a great success, and I retired a proud and fulfilled person. I regarded each member of this team as my colleague.

The first attached district nurse was Sister Margaret Ellis and she worked with us when the practice was a two-man partnership. John Lee and I found her to be a very caring person, and she and Dennis exchange Christmas cards with me still. I have occasionally bumped into them when I have been out and about. They came to a practice reunion party I held at my house in 2016.

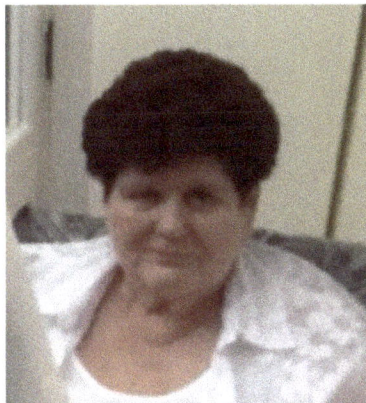

Margaret Ellis

The district nurse for the latter years of my working as a GP was Jackie Spencer. Time was no object with her. She was superb at terminal care and most popular. I had the fascinating experience of being her tutor for the Nurse Practitioner course run by Huddersfield University. This was a two-year part-time attachment with me. We undertook tutorials and joint surgeries. I really got to know her during that time. The course resulted in her obtaining a masters' degree. She became a nurse practitioner at the Knottingley Practice and specialised in mental health. Jackie worked closely with Margaret Wilkes. They were a great team.

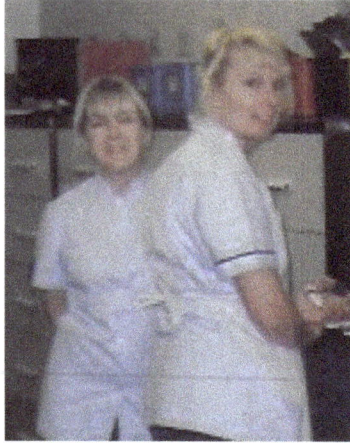

Margaret Wilkes (right) with Jackie Spencer

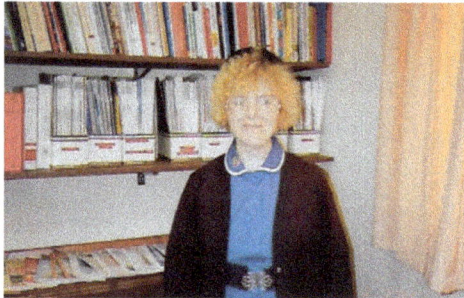

Jackie Spencer

Christine Hunter is the practice nurse in 2020. She started in 1988. That is over thirty years ago! I cannot praise Christine highly enough. Christine was supported by the practice to undertake a BSc (Hons) in nursing. She is an expert in asthma and diabetes and more besides.

She was a member of the practice group that was involved in a clinical supervision project for Huddersfield University. The results of the project were published for a conference in Brighton held in 2000. I would like to quote from that publication because it illustrates the depths of colleague relationships we were willing to explore.

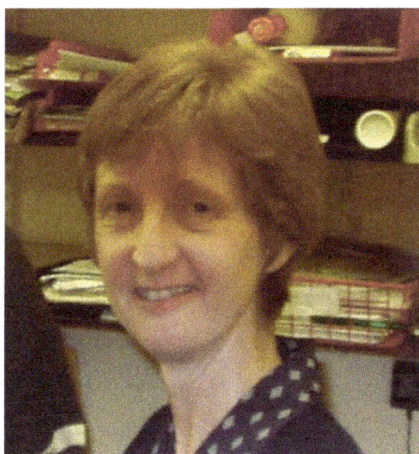

Christine Hunter

"The participants were all members of one General Practice team, who had worked together for many years. They consisted of: one District Nurse, one Health Visitor, one Practice Nurse, and one General Practitioner. (The GP was male, the nurses all female). The first two were employees of the local Community and Mental Health Trust, attached to the Practice. The Practice Nurse was an employee of the practice, at which the GP was a senior partner. The Practice was situated in an urban area, dominated by large council estates with a high level of deprivation. Of the three nurses, only the Practice Nurse had not experienced clinical supervision before, while the GP had experience of mentorship schemes. The Practice was noted for its involvement in a wide range of innovative schemes and research projects in primary care, and the participants had, in various combinations, worked together in the recent past on a number of these initiatives. Prior to the pilot, which ran for four 90-minute sessions, all participants attended two training sessions, each lasting two-and-a-half hours. These covered issues such as: definitions of clinical supervision; contracting and ground rules; the roles in group supervision; and reflective practice. The reflective cycle as described by Gibbs (1988) was offered as a framework for sessions, and this was adopted without alteration by the group."

"In her session as supervisee, the Practice Nurse was very evidently anxious about how the GP would respond to the issue she brought. When the GP responded positively, legitimising the Practice Nurse's concerns, the latter's relief was unmistakable. In the interview, she described her feelings at this point in the supervision session as 'elated'."

—King, Nigel, Roche, Tracy and Frost, Chrystal (2000) Diverse Identities, Common Purpose: Multi disciplinary Clinical Supervision in Primary Care. In: British Psychological Society Annual Occupational Psychology Conference, January 2000, Brighton, UK.

The practice nurse in this project was Christine, the health visitor Kathryn Padgett and the district nurse Jackie Spencer. I lost sleep the night before it was my turn to bring an issue to the group. That supervision experiment was career enhancing for me. Christine became a director of the company that owned the new surgery. I could always go to Christine and offload any worries I had. One interesting silly worry occurred to me just before I retired. Saying goodbye to some patients was difficult. Occasionally a woman patient would give me a goodbye kiss at the end of a consultation. On one occasion I was given a goodbye kiss in the street. Patients kissing doctors is not on! Each time this happened I told Christine! I have to say this did not happen often. It was pointed out, however, by Lynn Armstrong that one of these had had a crush on me for a year or more! How did Lynn know that?

Lynn Armstrong joined us as a receptionist in 1997. Eventually, she became one of the new healthcare assistants. This is a highly responsible job requiring good consultation skills and other skills such as taking blood, assessing blood pressures and more besides.

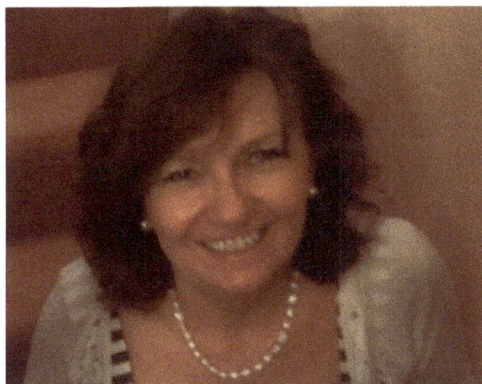

Lynn Armstrong

Some time in the 1990s I got interested in clinical audit. This interest was started by the GP Training Scheme course organiser, Jeffrey Ellis. GP trainees were expected to undertake a simple audit. Jeffrey asked me to do a half-day training session on audit with the GP trainees. I had no idea what clinical audit was all about. I read it up for the teaching session. Let me describe the process in the simplest way I can. It is a cycle of actions designed to make improvements. First one decides what one wants to improve – for example, the uptake of measles vaccination in children. Next one looks up the evidence as to what percentage of uptake is recommended. Then one measures the uptake. To improve the uptake, a change is then introduced, such as offering the vaccination in any surgery rather than just the children's clinic. The uptake is re-measured after, say, a year. If further improvement is wanted, another change can be introduced and so on. This is known as an audit cycle.

Kath, the practice manager, found that there was a grant available to pay for a short-term member of staff to do a project. We advertised for an audit administrator. One of the applicants was Richard Levitt. He was somewhat different from us all as he had a degree in classics from Oxford University and was trying to become a Methodist minister. I managed his work. He was very good at researching the literature and worked a couple of sessions a week for fifteen months.

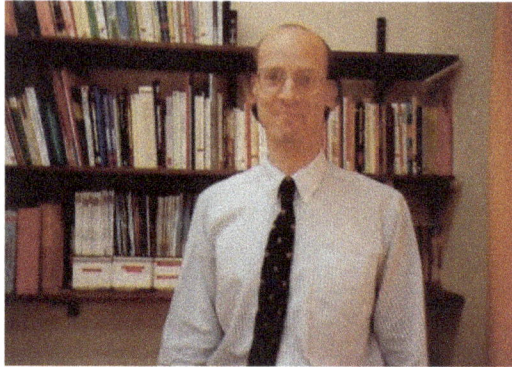

Richard Levitt

Kath retired as practice manager in 2000 and was replaced by Celia Burnhope, the practice development manager. Celia developed the practice and thus lived up to her job title. She negotiated an excellent contract that allowed us to have four and a half whole time equivalent GPs for just over 5000 patients. She oversaw the building of the huge new surgery with nineteen consulting rooms, rooms for health visitors and nurses, an education suite (including board room), a large common room, and a huge car park. She also negotiated successfully for us to have a significant increase in the number of nurses and administration staff. These negotiations were successful because the Primary Care Trust recognised what was needed in a deprived area like Airedale.

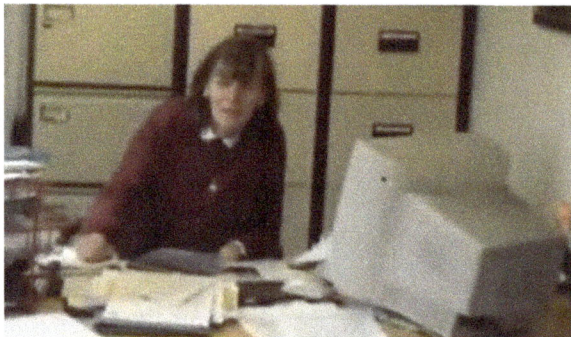

Celia Burnhope

Melanie Hanney was a practice nurse who undertook some groundbreaking work in triage. She now works in the Ophthalmology department at the Mid Yorkshire Trust.

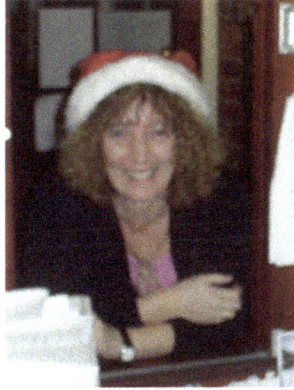

Melanie Hanney

Nicki Harrison worked as a practice nurse with Christine. She was appointed in 2000. She is a martial artist and Assistant Instructor at Sengoku Martial Arts based in Featherstone in West Yorkshire. I was wise and refrained from disagreeing with her to avoid my being thrown over her shoulder. She retired in 2020.

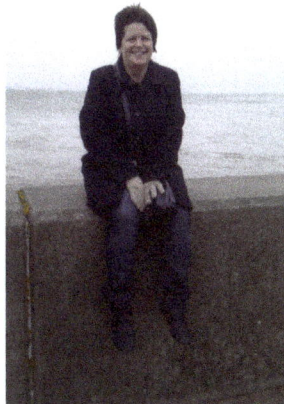

Nicki Harrison

Jane Herbert is a new appointment who worked with Jean Howarth when she was a practice administrator. I used to have a laugh with Jane when we remembered the occasion when she was on her knees in reception doing something and for some inexplicable reason slowly rolled over onto her left side. She did not hurt herself. This is the effect I have on people sometimes!

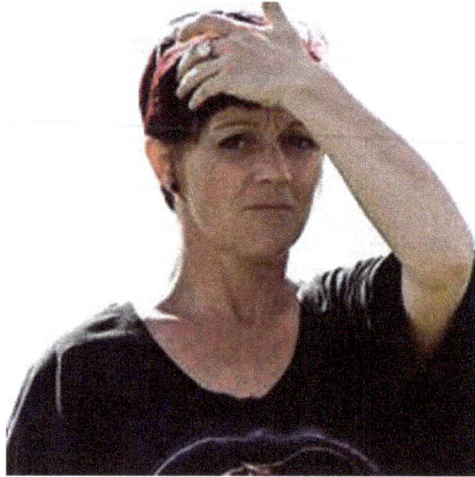

Jane Herbert

Four new receptionists were appointed in the latter years of my time at the practice: Rosemarie Rooker (2001–), Joanne Hainsworth (2001–2019), Susan Swift (2004–) and Julie Woodford (2001–). I retired in 2005 after winding down to three days a week of GP work. Sue Swift and Rosemarie Rooker are Facebook friends of mine. All four are great contributors to the team, and it is a shame I pulled back to three days a week and then retired relatively soon after they were appointed so that I did not get to know them better.

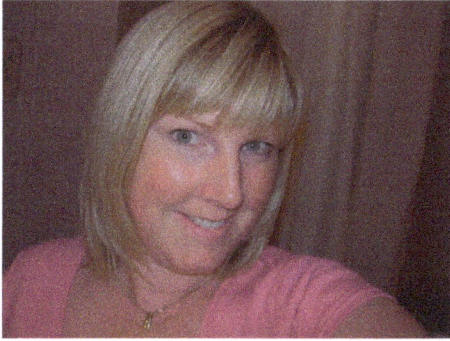

Sue Swift

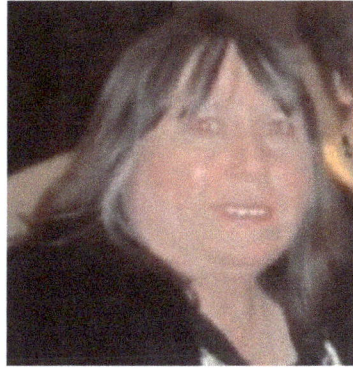

Rosemarie Rooker

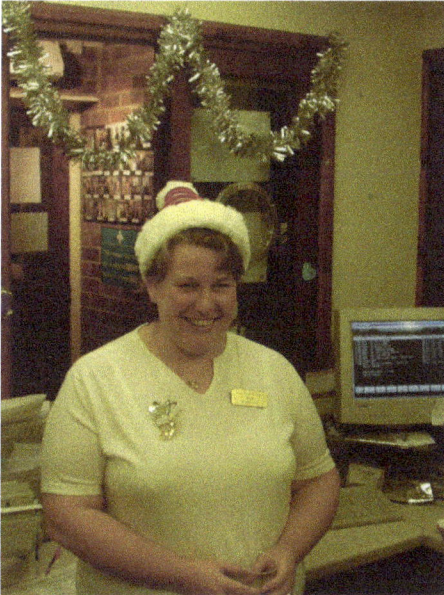

Julie Woolford

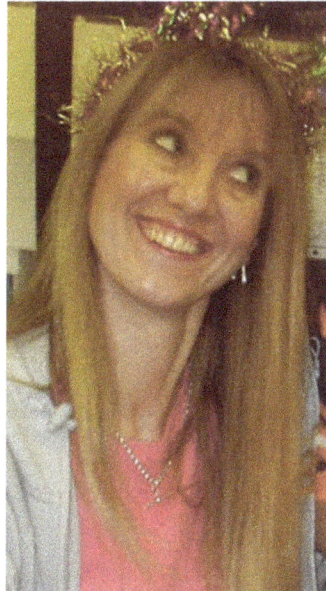

Joanne Hainsworth

Celia, the practice development manager, had a great talent for grabbing doctors and asking if they would consider working with us.

Sarah Baker had been working as an NHS manager in Leeds for a number of years, and I was asked to undertake the supervising of her familiarisation with general practice. It was easy for her to get up to speed. She became a partner and was great at suggesting and implementing change. She returned to a management job after being with us a relatively short time. She was an ordained Church of England minister and once asked me if I minded her praying with a patient. Of course, I did not. I said to her that I assumed that the prayers would not be with patients with sore throats. Sarah worked on reorganising our appointments system, and this was a great success. There is one partners' meeting I will not forget. I had spoken to two close GP colleagues (Liz Moulton and Grahame Smith) about the sabbatical breaks system each had in their practices. I wrote a brief paper on what I thought should happen in our practice. Sarah argued strongly against it and then said to me: "Nice try, Richard!" The points she made were spot on and the sabbatical break was never mentioned again. I did not mind at all.

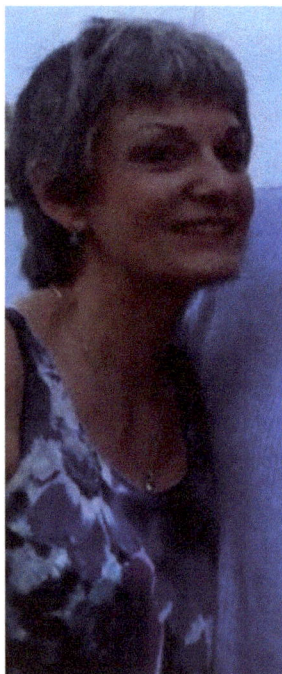

Sarah Baker

Celia set up a job share for Deborah Hewitt and Monica Smith. Debbie was my last full-time trainee, and I was thrilled when she became a partner in 2003 as I had got to know her well during her training attachment. She has a higher qualification in paediatric medicine. She is a quiet, modest and thoughtful person and during her attachment as a trainee always asked me interesting questions. We visited a patient who had been in the RAF in the Second World War. He had a handlebar moustache. She asked me why he had a moustache like that. I think it was tradition in the RAF. It is called after the handlebar of a bicycle.

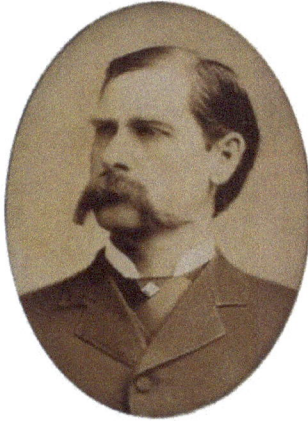

Wyatt Earp's moustache

I felt so lucky that Debbie decided to become a partner and make my last two years as a GP such a pleasure by joining a great team. She has been very kind and thoughtful towards me since my retirement and the death of my dear wife, Kath. She retired as a partner in early 2020 and works one day a week as a locum.

Monica was also a great partner and she became an appraiser. I worked with her on that as I ran the appraisal scheme for the Primary Care Trust. I was upset when, not so many years ago, Monica resigned to take up a job nearer where she lived in the York area. I met some of her York colleagues in November 2019. They spoke highly of her. She has become a trainer.

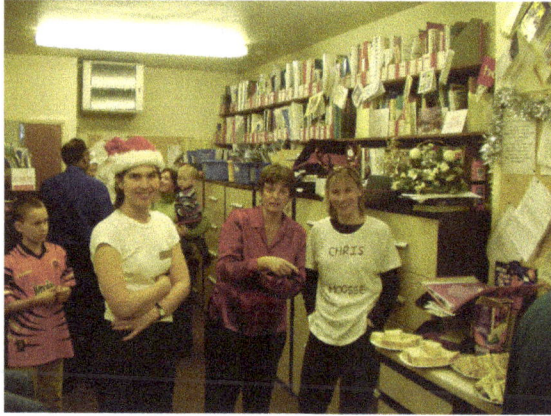

Deborah Hewitt, Sarah Baker and Monica Smith, left to right

Rosario Vega was a trainee with us and joined us as a salaried partner. Rosario was a fabulous partner and looked after the specialist care home which was nearby. There was a whole wing there which had patients with complex neurological diseases. Suddenly, after I retired, the practice was deprived of a huge amount of money by the managing authority. Rosario was made redundant, as was a member of the administrative staff. Rosario moved from Tieve Tara to be an equity partner in a practice in Pontefract. Both she and her husband are Facebook friends of mine.

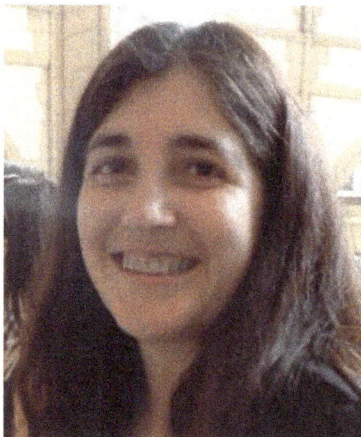

Rosario Vega

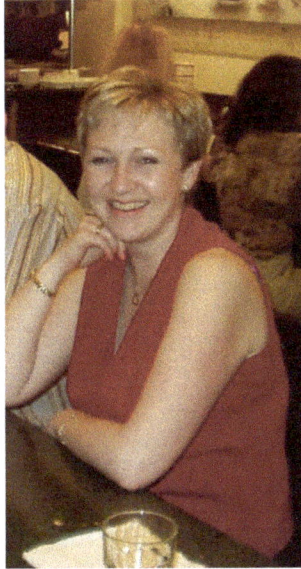

Samantha Kaye

Samantha Kaye was employed as a receptionist/administrator. This again was in my latter years. I mention her just after Rosario because she was the other member of staff made redundant by the financial cut I just mentioned. If I had still been there, I would have been incandescent with anger and taken legal advice and appealed.

Graham Bond joined us and was a trainer and expert in diabetes. He retired not so many years ago. I did not work with him for very long before I retired. It was good that the practice had two trainers – Graham and Anne.

Joti Agarwol lived in Manchester and commuted to and from the practice daily, starting later in the morning than the rest of us. He was a partner for only a few years and was one of the directors of the company (Motorstep Ltd.) that owned the fabric of the surgery. One memory of him is the professional joystick he used on his Flight Simulator for his computer. I think he had a degree in maths. Celia, Deborah, Anne, Monica, Christine and I were the other directors of Motorstep Ltd. The company was sold round about 2008/9 right in the middle of the Libor crisis. It was a nightmare for me, and I vowed I would not be involved in that sort of business ever again. However, we directors made a good profit, and I spent my share on a new car for me and Kath.

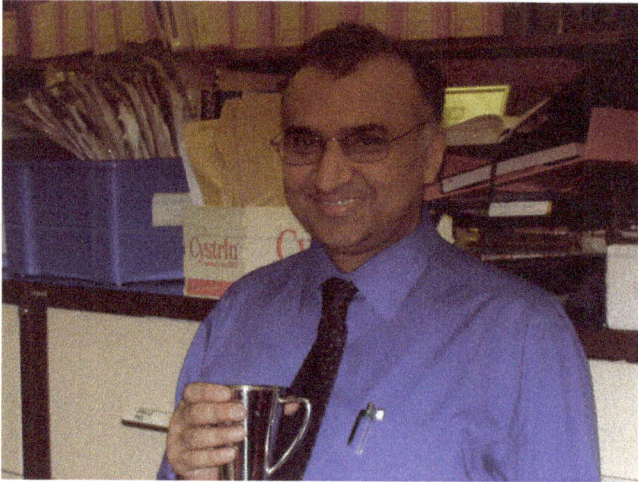

Joti Agarwol

When I started writing this chapter, I entitled it "Partners and Staff". Halfway through I realised, as I have mentioned above, what a fantastic group of people we were. I renamed the chapter "Colleagues".

To work in such a difficult area as Airedale required a very special team. It is the memory of this team that has helped make reflections on my professional and private life in Airedale a joy.

Chapter 5 – Associates

Whom do I regard as associates? They are the solicitor and accountant who are vitally important for any general practice; pharmacists; an insurance broker; hospital consultants; managers of secondary care (the hospitals, social services, etc.); managers of the financing of general practice; the undertaker and others.

My definition of an associate of Tieve Tara Surgery/Medical Centre is someone in these organisations who became a friend of the practice and who gave honest advice and counsel. So, some of the associates became my friends in the fullness of time. Others had close professional relationships with my mother and father. I developed a special relationship with some of them.

Maurice Smith was the solicitor for my parents and the practice. His family became friends of my family. I sought advice from Maurice when I was a final year medical student. I had received a third endorsement on my driving licence and was due to be disqualified. Maurice gave me good advice on writing a statement regarding mitigating circumstances. At the court case, the statement resulted in a very low fine, but I was disqualified from driving for six months.

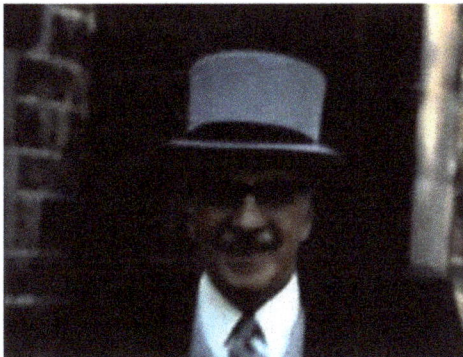

Maurice Smith

Maurice and Muriel's son, Christopher, was a close school friend of mine. He became a successful solicitor in London, and we meet there occasionally for lunch.

Another school friend, Peter Box, worked in the Castleford office and was an expert in wills and inheritance. He dealt with my mother's will. Peter's family were also friends of my parents. He was a successful leader of Wakefield Council for twenty-one years and was awarded the CBE a few years ago. He retired recently to become chair of Welcome to Yorkshire. I have to walk behind him at certain official functions as my MBE is a lower award! It is amazing what happens with friends with the passage of the years. It was obvious that the firm should be our solicitor when we arrived in Castleford in 1978. Maurice had retired by then.

The first solicitor Kath and I used when we bought the house and surgery from my mother was Richard Pinto. He was the senior partner in the Castleford office. In the very early days, setting up the practice with Kath, I was definitely a bit crazy. I received what I thought was a hefty bill from Mr. Pinto. One of my friends told me to pay him in cash as a protest. I took the money in to him personally. He simply took it from me, counted it slowly, and gave me a receipt. I felt a complete fool.

I became involved with the Wakefield Dyslexia Association, and its secretary was Julia Dale. Her husband, Brian, was a solicitor in Wakefield. Brian was the practice solicitor for many years from the early 1980s until his untimely death from cancer. He was also my and Kath's personal solicitor. It was a tradition with GPs to have the same solicitor for both personal matters and the business. Brian was a gentle, quiet and wise man. Julia and I exchange Christmas cards.

In the latter years, the practice solicitor was Roy Cusworth of Beaumont Legal in Wakefield. This is a massive firm, and Roy is the senior partner. The firm has a great reputation. Roy occasionally came to work in his Rolls Royce (or was it a Bentley?). During the financial crisis in 2008/9, he started coming to work in his Range Rover. He told me he felt it was rather tasteless to drive a big car at this time of such anxiety in the workplace!

He dealt with the legal aspects of building the last huge surgery extension, which was completed in 2004. He also set up a company called Motorstep Ltd. There were seven directors, and the company owned the fabric and fixtures of the building as I mentioned in Chapter 4. I think it was just at the start of the financial crisis in 2008/9 that the directors decided to sell Motorstep to a property company. It sold for well over one million pounds, and after significant expenses, each director received their share of the profit. The sale took place during the Libor crisis when interest charges were fluctuating widely. (It was discovered later that the Libor rates were being fixed in a fraudulent manner.) That time involved Roy working very late and at weekends and Kath and I being asked to fax through signed documents late in the evenings. I would never like to experience anything like that again despite making some easy money.

Regarding large solicitors' bills, I would have needed a truck to take pound coins to Beaumont Legal to pay their fee for selling Motorstep Ltd. The bill was a significant number of tens of thousands of pounds. It was worth every penny to me. Roy was indeed a wise friend of the practice and has been a wise advisor to me and Kath. His firm is my solicitor now.

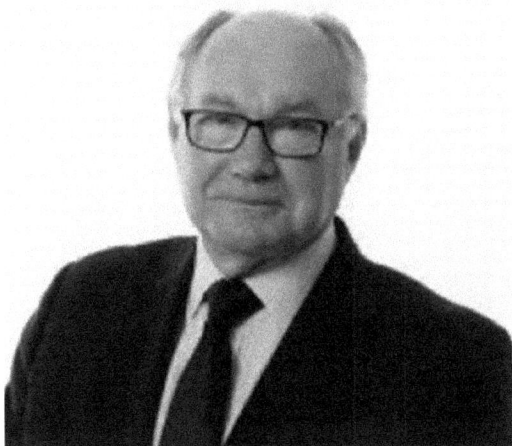

Roy Cusworth

My parents' personal and general practice accountant was Charles Davison. Charles and his wife, Doris, were family friends of my parents. He worked for Hansons Accountants in Castleford. He became our practice accountant in 1978 and, of course, completed the tax returns for Kath and me. Charles did the first year accounts when the practice made a loss. Charles was also made joint power of attorney with me for my mother. I asked her why she had decided to include Charles. She said she wanted someone she could trust! This was typical of my mother's sense of humour. Or was it?

Soon after John Lee became a partner, he introduced Kath and me to an accountant with whom he had been at school. Nick Cudmore became the practice's accountant in the early 1980s and has remained so ever since. Of course, he was my and Kath's accountant, and he and his colleagues (Duncan & Toplis, Louth) continue to prepare my personal tax returns and give me advice. Nick quickly realised I was pretty hopeless at reading balance sheets etc. He always explained the practice's annual accounts in a way we understood. He came all the way from Louth in Lincolnshire and distance seemed no object for him.

Nick has a great sense of humour. He once kicked off a meeting with: "We will start with Richard giving a short talk on the capital account." I think I nearly know what this is. Once, on his arrival for a meeting, Nick noticed one of the trainees, Paco Fernandez, on his knees on the floor in reception surrounded by lots of cards on which he was writing. At the meeting, we explained that Paco was Spanish and had difficulty understanding patients' addresses on the phone when a home visit was being requested. This actually could have been a dangerous situation. Nick commented that if Paco did not get through his assessment to become a GP, he could always become a taxi driver.

A year or so ago I went out for lunch with Nick and his wife. I will certainly stay with his firm. He is a fantastic accountant. He retired in 2020.

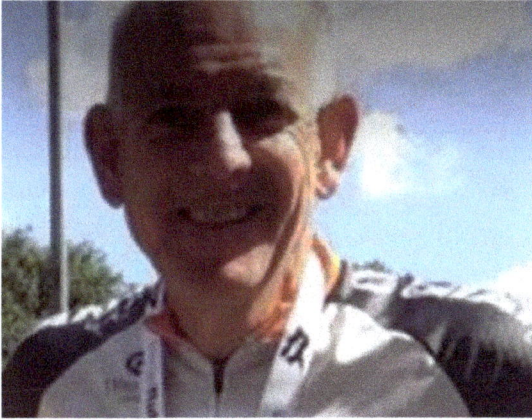

Nick Cudmore

In the early days from 1978 we used Tim Powell for insurance matters for both the practice and our house and cars. He and his wife, Pat, were friends of mine in Cheltenham. He was an insurance broker. He was somewhat addicted to betting on the horses. In the early 1980s Kath and I went to Barbados for the new year with seventeen friends from Cheltenham, including Tim and Pat. I was the "medical officer" for the group, which included small children. There was some illness in the group while we were there. Tim developed gastroenteritis shortly before we were about to fly home and he became seriously anxious about the flight. I had some Valium in my medical kit, which I gave him. He got home OK.

When I decided to leave Cheltenham, I held a party. I set up a roulette table and bought a green eye shade for Tim for his use as croupier. We raised quite a lot of money for charity, but it could have easily gone the other way.

On an occasion when they were staying with us, Tim and I went down to the Fryston Hotel, the local pub frequented mainly by miners and their families. It was a rough pub and lots of the patients went there. The barmaid that evening was a patient of mine. Tim was an obvious newcomer. She asked him whether he was a policeman or from social security. When he answered that he was not, she said, "Have a drink."

Tim maintained that he could obtain insurance for anything. That included the possibility of a toy boat sinking in the bath. He died quite young from a stroke.

The local pharmacists were associates. When I was a child, Harold Carter was the pharmacist at Timothy Whites in the Magnet area of Airedale. (That area is called after the name of one of the pubs.) Harold and his wife were friends of my parents. They often came to the house for a social occasion and I remember my mother playing cards with them. That was the only chemist's shop in the area in the 1950s.

In the early 1960s another pharmacy was established not so far away in the new estate, Ferry Fryston. The pharmacist was Michael Elbogen. He was an astute businessman and eventually the Timothy Whites pharmacy could not compete. I believe that this was because Michael kept a huge stock of medicines. He bought out the Timothy Whites shop and business. So Michael ran two pharmacies for a while until he eventually closed the one in the estate. He was very friendly with my parents. In 1978 when I came back to Airedale, he told me I would never make it. He took the side of my competitors, for that is what my fellow local GPs were when I was building up the business. I actually did what Michael did and provided a service that the patients liked. The customer comes first. He and I fell out for a while, but in the end he was big enough to admit he was wrong, and Kath and I were invited for dinner in his apartment in Leeds. We made it up completely. He sold his pharmacy to Lloyds when he retired.

There was a pharmacist in Castleford town I want to mention who was not an associate of the practice but was a great character. He was called Stanley Z. Jackson. He patented a cough medicine called Cab Drivers' Linctus. He made a huge amount of money out of this. It is a great name for a cough medicine. I wonder if cab drivers have a particular problem with coughing. From 1995, GPs were not allowed to prescribe this anymore.

We used to invite Mike Freeman to our Christmas "fuddle" (drinks and bites to eat in the surgery). We invited him simply because he was a nice and decent man. He owned a pharmacy in

Castleford town. It is interesting that, like me, these three pharmacists are Jewish.

The undertaker in Airedale in my childhood days was Norman Dean. He became a patient of the practice when I returned to Airedale. I was looked after by a live-in nanny called Mrs. Price. Every Sunday, Mrs. Price went to visit her daughter Maud in Castleford town. Norman Dean used to take her there and back in one of his huge black funeral limousines. I remember him occasionally taking her in the hearse. She sat in the front, of course.

After Norman, the main undertaker in Airedale was Trevor Morritt. Kath and I really got on with him. If ever we were in the congregation at a funeral that he was managing, he would give us a big wink as he passed us. If a deceased person was to be cremated, two GPs had to examine the body and complete a form to state that there were no reasons for the body not to be cremated. We were mainly looking for foul play. Once, when I approached a body I was to examine, I noticed there was a pencil affixed between the nose and the side of the coffin. I asked Trevor why this was. He explained that when they were carrying the body into the chapel of rest, the head bumped into the entrance door and the nose was bent. He was trying to straighten it before the relatives came to view.

James, the son of one of our best friends, Geof, was a medical student at St Mary's Hospital Medical School in London. He stayed with us for a week's attachment in general practice. He spent a day with Trevor, who showed him everything including visiting behind the scenes at Pontefract Crematorium. James was so impressed with that educational experience that I did the same thing with Trevor at a later date. It was indeed fascinating. I was so impressed by the reverence shown towards the coffins and ashes by the staff working at the crematorium. They showed us two urns of ashes, one of a 20-stone person and another of an 8-stone person, and asked us which of the ashes was the heavier. The answer was they were of nearly identical weights because it is only the bones that remain as ashes.

Trevor, his wife and son and his parents were patients of the practice and I mainly dealt with them. Trevor died aged in his fifties. It was a surreal and awful experience for us to attend his funeral.

The undertaker based in Castleford town is Charles Ashton & Son. Mr. Ashton does not wink at me at funerals but always comes up to me and shakes my hand. I think he is measuring me up. At the end of a funeral in St. Joseph's Church, Pontefract, in April 2019, the hearse was waiting to set off to the crematorium. As I passed, Mr. Ashton asked the driver to get out to meet me. The driver was Mr. Ashton's son and partner. It was embarrassing for me in front of all the people but a friendly act of the Ashtons.

When I went to the chapel of rest at Ashton's to complete a cremation form, Charles Ashton always asked: "Would you like to use my desk?" Then he would lead me to a coffin and the papers were completed with my resting them on a coffin lid. GPs were paid well for completing these forms as it was quite a responsibility. They were paid by the undertaker, who billed the relations of the deceased. For many years in the early days, the pay was in cash and this income was not generally declared to the Inland Revenue. This avoidance was rife all over the UK. It was nicknamed "ash cash". However, the taxman caught up with this in the end.

There were people in the administrative and management bodies of the NHS that were associates of the practice. There were so many re-organisations of the NHS that the names of these bodies changed frequently. The Area Health Authority seemed to be around quite a long time. It managed the hospitals and more besides. If you want to know about NHS management history, have a look at this article in the Health Service Journal: https://www.hsj.co.uk/organisations/kings-fund/nhs-management-history-milestones/5020517.article.

Dr. Colin Pollock was a public health consultant and was a great friend of Wakefield District GPs. He was the first person I came across in the NHS management system who appreciated properly that our medical practice in Airedale, Castleford, was looking after seriously deprived people. He even arranged for one of his junior colleagues to do a study of this situation.

I worked with Colin and others on the Local Medical Committee's Professional Support Group. This looked into situations where GPs were alleged to be poorly performing, behaving oddly or ill. He was such a great help to us when Dr. Bazaz, our partner, became ill. Kath and I socialised with the Pollocks for a while and I have always kept in touch. Colin and I are Facebook friends. We met in 2018 for a coffee at my house.

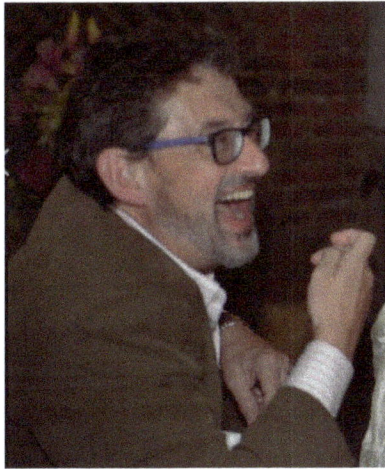

Colin Pollock

Wendy Pearson was the finance manager at the Health Authority when the system of fundholding for GPs was running. I objected to fundholding on ethical grounds. Practices were given a fund and if they underspent, that saving could be spent on the practice. I believed that if one built an extension from fundholding savings, then the GPs owned that extension and could cash in on retirement. At the same time, one could create a decent underspend by not referring patients to consultants, doing fewer investigations, prescribing less and more cheaply, etc. We resisted fundholding but eventually were forced to join the system when some of our attached staff were being taken away to work in fundholding practices. We were small and had to join with another small practice in South Elmsall. The two practices were about 10 miles apart. How crazy! The senior partner there was Dr. Douglas

Diggle, and we were of like minds regarding fundholding. We had to attend regular meetings with Wendy to discuss our financial status. The best thing about those meetings was that Wendy was a charming person to meet and tolerated us politely. I am sure she rumbled that we were clueless about fundholding. Douglas and I did not really know what she was talking about regarding the finances of this fundholding system. We simply nodded a lot.

I used to tell my colleagues in the Wakefield medical world that I had once spent a weekend with Wendy in Madrid. She and I were members of a group that went to Madrid to assess and recruit GPs from Spain. This was when I was working for the Primary Care Trust after I retired. Wendy was a director in that trust. It really was through my work in postgraduate GP education that I was in that visiting party. She too is a Facebook friend now.

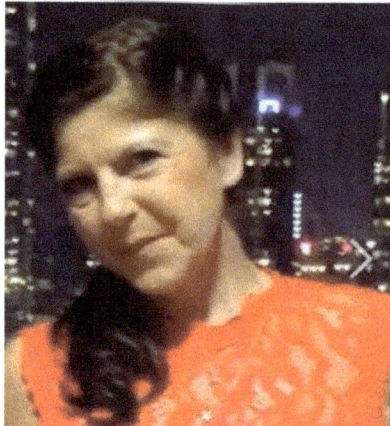

Wendy Pearson

Another Facebook friend is Andrea Robinson. She eventually became the director of nursing and operations for the Primary Care Trust. Her very successful career journey included her appointment as the chief executive of the Wakefield Health Authority. There was a coup while she was on maternity leave, and when she returned to work that job had been taken by another. That might not have been exactly how it happened, but it is how I saw it.

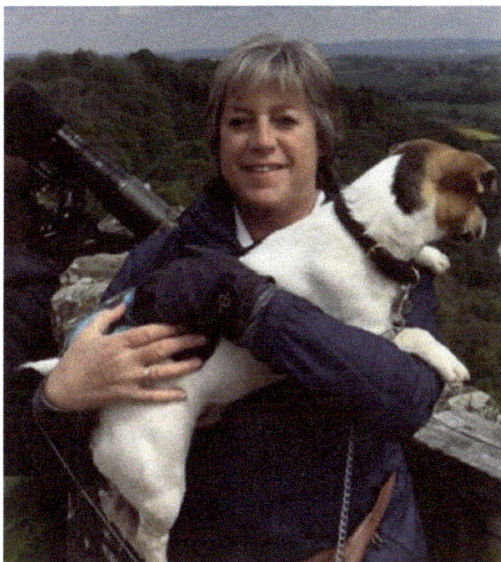

Andrea Robinson (Hopkins)

Shelagh Taylor was a health visitor by background. We met her when she had a management role working for the Health Authority and, later, the Primary Care Trust. She was known as Julia at work. I never got to grips with why this was so. She became the facilitator for the Wakefield area for practices wanting to undertake the King's Fund Organisational Audit. With her help and that of an administrator employed by the practice, Carolyn Cranton, we were recognised in the mid-1990s as achieving the standards of that audit. It involved very hard work by the whole team in writing and understanding a whole host of procedures and policies. Shelagh and her husband, Paul, became good friends of mine and Kath's. We regularly met several times a year for more than twenty years and were joined by other friends. We would each bring a CD and play a couple of tracks of music accompanied by a bite to eat. We called these meetings Desert Island Discs. Shelagh died from cancer in the summer of 2019. It is so sad that five of the original group are no longer with us. They will be listening to heavenly music now.

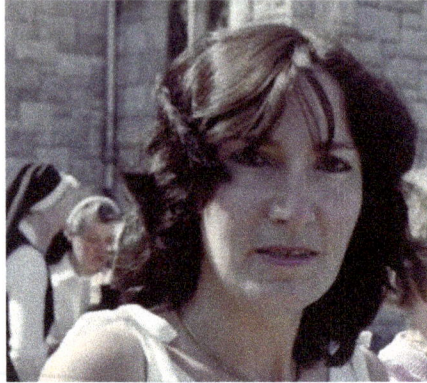

Shelagh Taylor

There were some GPs and consultants working in the Wakefield district whom I would regard as associates of Tieve Tara Surgery/Medical Centre. These professional relationships developed over many years, and I still meet one or two of them now. I could have written what follows in the chapter on colleagues, but all the consultants we worked with were colleagues.

My parents, particularly my mother, held consultants in very high regard. I think it was a bit of a disappointment to my mother that I never became a consultant!

At the start of the NHS in 1948, a system of consultant domiciliary visits was introduced. A GP could request a consultant to visit a patient at home when a second opinion was required. This opinion often resulted in the patient being looked after at home or as an out- patient rather than being admitted to hospital. In the days before I left home, my mother or father would meet the consultant in our house. They would have a cup of tea (or a glass of whiskey for one of them) and discuss the patient, current affairs and holidays – and not necessarily in that order. They would then visit the patient together. This system was still in operation in the early part of my GP career. It was a great way of establishing closer relationships between consultants and GPs. However, as we all got busier, the consultant would visit alone and phone up the GP with his or her opinion. They were paid a fee for doing such a visit and extra for undertaking an ECG recording.

There were three consultants whom I regarded as very good associates of mine. These were John Turner (general physician and cardiologist), Peter Howe (obstetrician and gynaecologist) and Jean Wharton (gastroenterologist). My relationship with the first two developed because of the professional relationship built up with each of them by my parents, particularly my mother. Jean was brought up in Castleford and was friends with my sisters, Dorothy and Gerry, and came to Tieve Tara house to play when they were children. She was a relatively new consultant at Pontefract Hospital.

John Turner was a one-off. He, like many consultants, enjoyed the rewards of private practice and the outings and meals paid for by pharmaceutical companies. He once featured in a BBC Panorama programme about doctors and drug companies. He was filmed enjoying a meal on the Orient Express on the way to Venice!

One of my friends, who was a patient, phoned me one Sunday morning. He had chest pain. I dealt with this in a very poor way and taking big risks as you will see. I phoned up John Turner and he said he would see my friend at his home. My friend was well off and could afford such a private appointment. I told my friend to stop off at our local off-licence and buy Dr. Turner a bottle of something, which he did. It was, as I suspected, a heart attack and he was admitted to hospital. Of course, I should have advised him not to drive, although Dr. Turner was also aware he was driving.

John Turner was a close colleague of my parents. When my mother developed diabetes, he dealt with it by advice over the phone. To my knowledge she never consulted anyone face to face about her diabetes apart from an ophthalmic surgeon. I was working in London when she developed diabetes and I wrote to Dr. Turner about my mother's drinking too much alcohol. I asked if he could have a word with her about that. He never replied to my letter. He was the only consultant my mother invited to her retirement party held in Tieve Tara house. My job was to serve the drinks. The main drink was a champagne cocktail. This was a lethal cocktail of a sugar lump covered with brandy and then the glass topped up with champagne. After several of these, Dr. Turner said to me: "Richard, don't you think that with the state of present society it is difficult to get through life on less than half a bottle of spirits a day?" I had no reply to that! That was his reply to my letter.

Another remarkable thing about Dr. Turner was that he visited a patient of ours fortnightly and sometimes more frequently. The patient had a serious complication from a drug and was virtually bed-ridden. That drug was eventually withdrawn from use. I have no idea whether this was a paid-for private consultation but, again, the patient could afford that. The patient invited Dr. Turner, me and our wives for an evening meal in the Wentbridge House Hotel near Pontefract. I did not think the patient would be well enough to get through the evening, but he did. However, that was at the expense of his health for about a week afterwards. He eventually died a couple of years later. There were not many at the funeral, but I and Dr. Turner were there. After the funeral, standing on the steps outside the door of the church, I asked him why he did all those visits to our patient. He simply said, "The NHS owed him."

John Turner was a great cricket fan. It was rumoured (and I am sure this is not true!) that he occasionally cancelled his outpatient clinic if there was a good match on at Headingley, Leeds. I have mentioned the Box family more than once in this book. Dr. Turner was a good friend of George Box, the barber. George also loved cricket and they once went off on a holiday together to watch some matches in Barbados. Dr. Turner died at Headingley Cricket Ground. A fitting end, I think.

Peter Howe was another consultant who became fond of my mother. Peter's wife, Margaret, dealt with his gynaecology private practice. My mother sent quite a few patients to him privately and this involved her phoning Margaret. A fellow GP and my friend, Grahame Smith, got to know Peter when he was the anaesthetist for some of Peter's operating sessions. Kath and I first met Peter socially at a party at Grahame and Caroline's house. Another time, when my sister Dorothy was staying with us, we went to a dinner which was to raise money for a charity Peter and Margaret supported. My sister sat next to Peter and you might have thought it was a highlight of her life the way she talked about sitting next to a gynaecologist. It reminded me of how the late Joan Rivers, the comedienne, used to talk about her gynaecologist all the time.

The chief executive of Pontefract Infirmary, Tony Woolgar, perceived that Peter had a performance problem. I was amazed when Peter phoned me at home one evening and asked me to write a letter of support. Of course, I did this. One time when I was in Pontefract Infirmary Postgraduate Centre, Tony Woolgar asked me to come into a small kitchen with him and he closed the door behind us. He said that only I and Peter's next-door neighbour had written in. I have always believed that Peter was a good man and a very competent and careful surgeon. Peter suffered a major stroke and he and others put this down to the pressure he was under regarding his work. Grahame and I occasionally visited him in his retirement after his stroke. Margaret looked after him like gold and that was very hard work. He required a hoist to get in and out of bed and other significant aids. Peter's condition slowly deteriorated such that he could understand what was being said but did not speak. On the last visit we made, I asked him whether he remembered my mother. He said "Yes, Gerda." That was the only thing he said while we were there. The funeral was well attended by hospital and other of his colleagues. I attend St. Joseph's Church, Pontefract, and it is lovely to occasionally meet Margaret there and have a brief chat.

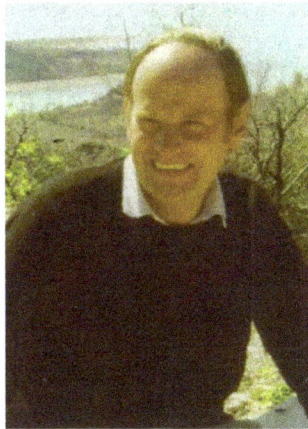

Peter Howe

Jean Wharton was a consultant gastroenterologist. She was brought up in Castleford and was a friend of my sisters, Gerry and Dorothy. She came to the house to play, sometimes with her brother. Maureen Wood, the daughter of Mrs. McGrath (the housekeeper at that time) used to look after her brother. Jean lived in the village of Burghwallis, and Kath and I went for lunch there. I went to Jean's funeral. My memory of that funeral is of one of the hymns. It was "All things bright and beautiful". The situation was a first for me. I stood up and sang the hymn with the consultant physician and my friend, Mick Peake, on my right and the chief executive of the hospital, Tony Woolgar, on my left.

The only associates I am in touch with now are Nick Cudmore, Wendy Pearson, Andrea Robinson and Colin Pollock, who are Facebook friends of mine.

I will digress somewhat to end this chapter. It is apparent to me that there are two personality types I see in my friends and colleagues. Those who appreciate Facebook, Twitter, WhatsApp, etc. and those who think they are a bad thing. An invasion of privacy etc. Some feel it is beneath them to use these social media or that they are too old.

One of my teachers at University College London gave the second Reith lectures and wrote a book based on those lectures. My favourite quote from the book is:

> "Whether we like it or not, we can be sure that societies that use to the full the new techniques of communication, by better language and by better machines, will eventually replace those that do not."

> —YOUNG J Z (1951) Doubt and Certainty in Science. A biologist's reflections on the brain. Oxford University Press.

The machines mentioned, of course, include computers and the printing presses used to produce newspapers and magazines. Darwin's theory of evolution, which embraces "survival of the fittest" (i.e. the strongest), has been modified by J. Z. Young to "survival of the best communicators".

In my opinion, Facebook is a marvellous method of keeping in touch with people and establishing and maintaining relationships in a different – but equally significant – way to face-to-face communication.

Chapter 6 – Training

In 1973 I became a GP without any special training for that discipline. For three years I undertook research in Physiology (on human temperature regulation) in a laboratory at The London Hospital Medical College. I only saw one patient during that time. That was to look at a defect in his temperature system. Quite honestly, when I started as a GP, I was dangerous. I had to learn quickly. From 1981, a compulsory year in general practice was introduced for new GPs and then, from August 1982, there was a three-year period of mandatory training to become a principal. (Hasler, J. C. History of vocational training for general practice: the 1970s and 1980s. J. Royal College of GPs, 1989 338–341).

I am sure that most members of the general public are unaware of the process that results in a competent general practitioner and how GPs keep up to date. I can describe the system up to my retirement in some detail.

In the early 1980s, I had an ambition for Tieve Tara Surgery to become a training practice and for me to become a trainer of prospective GPs.

There were two streams to be addressed before I would be able to work in my practice as a trainer.

First, there were rules to be obeyed and standards to be attained for a practice to be approved. Second, I had to be assessed and approved to be a suitable person and teacher to become a trainer. Achieving these two elements was daunting.

The training of GPs was managed, at first, by the Regional Advisor in General Practice and its education committee. This body was known as the Yorkshire Deanery. The offices were in Leeds. It was the responsibility of the Deanery and its Advisor in General Practice, to approve a practice by an inspection and approve a GP as a trainer by a variety of methods of assessment.

The most daunting task for the practice was a target that all patient records should have a summary of past and present medical problems written out on a card. (Later these were computerised.) Dr. John Lee, my medical partner, worked really hard with me on this. It involved slowly going through each patient's medical records. At one point we experimented and paid a retired health visitor to write summaries. Her summaries were as good as any doctor's. The summaries had to be kept up to date.

The trainee GP had to have a fully equipped consulting room to him or herself. This was achieved after the first extension.

The practice had to have a comprehensive library of reference books and magazines. There was a recommended list of these produced by the Deanery. We brought in loads of books from our homes and lent them permanently to the practice. Of course, we had to buy the books we did not possess. I did hear of a practice that borrowed a whole library of books from a training practice for the assessment day.

A timetable was produced which showed protected time for education for both the trainee and trainer. It was not allowed for either to be the on-call doctor at the time of a tutorial. Tutorials could not be interrupted.

The practice had to own a video camera and a monitor. This was so that videos of patient consultations with the trainee could be made and discussed with the trainer. The development of good consulting skills was of prime importance. Trainers also videoed their consultations. These videos were not only used to teach trainees but were also submitted to the Deanery as part of the reaccreditation of training status every two or three years. Many years after I had been appointed as a trainer, I became a video assessor for the Deanery.

Part of my training to be a trainer involved regularly attending trainers' workshops. These were held once a month in either an evening or an afternoon and were managed by the course organiser. The Yorkshire Deanery was divided into geographical areas, each of which had a hospital, a postgraduate education centre and a course organiser. My area was Pontefract. Wakefield was our neighbouring vocational training area. Most course organisers were also trainers; Susan Butler, a close colleague, became the first course organiser who was not. She argued that the course organiser was an administrative post, and she was right. The course organiser was responsible for the continuing education and support of the trainers (the workshop) and also for a weekly half-day release teaching afternoon for the trainees.

I did not feel at all welcome at the first trainers' workshop. This was mainly due to my being regarded as a bit of an intruder by the other trainers, whom I did not know well. At these meetings, difficulties with trainees as well as teaching methods were addressed. The course organiser for Pontefract was Jeffrey Ellis, and he was most helpful in my becoming a trainer.

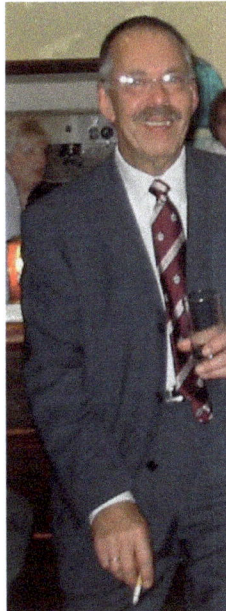

Jeffrey Ellis, VTS Course Organiser, Pontefract

There was also a course put on by the Deanery called the "O" course. I have never found out what the "O" stood for. The course was a mixture of teaching and assessment of us as potential trainers. The course was residential, over three nights, and took place in Ripon in a large house in the extensive grounds of the

College of Ripon and York St. John, a teacher training college. The house, called the Short Course Centre, had a few bedrooms but these were for what I called the "high and mighty" – the tutors. I stayed with a history teacher and his family in their house nearby. I became one of the "high and mighty" many years later.

There were about twenty prospective trainers from Yorkshire on that O course. I knew two of them – Geof Slater and Douglas Diggle. The managing tutor for the course was Martin Rogers. It took me a day and a half to realise he was not a doctor! He was a man of faith and an educationalist.

Part of the course involved splitting us into small groups who went to breakout rooms with a task. Sometimes we got to the breakout room and had no idea what Martin had been talking about or what we were to do. Douglas could not stand it and left early. He never became a trainer. Geof and I became totally paranoid as the time went on as we knew the tutors were watching and listening to us, even at mealtimes. One evening we escaped to the students' bar but after a couple of pints thought the barman was a course organiser in disguise. Geof was a Geordie with a great sense of humour. He died not so many years ago.

I knew that the Oxford region had made it mandatory that trainers should have the higher general practice qualification, the MRCGP (Membership of the Royal College of General Practitioners). I decided to take that examination and failed the first time. I should not have argued with the oral examiner. I still think he was wrong about the point I was making. I passed the second time. It was many years after I had become a trainer that passing the MRCGP was mandatory for becoming a trainer in Yorkshire. (For a few years now, passing the MRCGP has been part of the final assessment of a trainee becoming a principal in general practice.)

As I mentioned earlier, there were two parts to the final assessment of becoming a new trainer. The first was a detailed inspection of the practice, which also involved my being assessed. Before that official inspection, the course organiser, Jeffrey Ellis, did a run-through. We had a coffee in our kitchen, and he smoked a significant number of my cigarettes. When I first met Jeff, I thought he was somewhat formidable, but he was one of the best course organisers I have come across and also most supportive of me. The formal assessment of the practice was undertaken by the deputy regional advisor (later to become director), Jamie Bahrami. He had a reputation for being a stickler for the rules, and I was extremely nervous of meeting him. I was not quite up to the target for the medical records summary and came clean rather than trying to get away with it. He was happy with that, and there was a further simple check on this later. You will see, later in the chapter, that Jamie became one of my medical heroes and I ended up working very closely with him. We are still in contact.

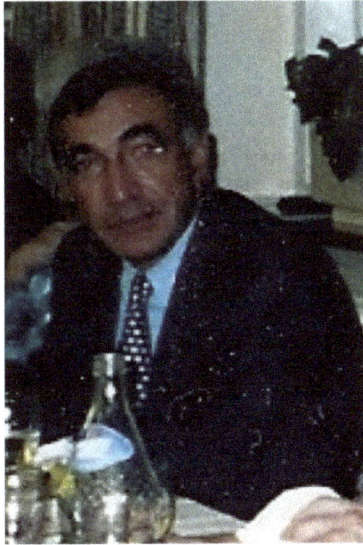

Dr. Jamie Bahrami. Director of Postgraduate General Practice Education, The Yorkshire Deanery

The final stage of my assessment was a daunting interview by about ten people. I got through that, but it made me sweat. We applicants all knew that one of the questions that might be asked was which books one had in the practice library. One candidate came out of his interview and was shocked that not only was he asked which books were in his library but also if he had read any of them! I was accepted as a trainer and was thrilled.

Trainees for general practice (later known as GP registrars) had to undertake three years of attachments, usually in six-month blocks. Two of the six-month periods were in different general practices. The other four blocks were in relevant and approved hospital jobs such as paediatrics, obstetrics, accident and emergency, etc.

Spending six months in a one-to-one teaching relationship with a fellow doctor was a privilege. I learned such a lot from each one of them and have some wonderful memories of that time. Of course, I had to swat up on topics for tutorials, which was a great learning experience for me. I am sure most of the trainees enjoyed working at Tieve Tara Surgery. At one point, Kath and the practice team organised a party to celebrate an award the practice had been given. As part of that celebration, unbeknown to me, many past trainees were invited.

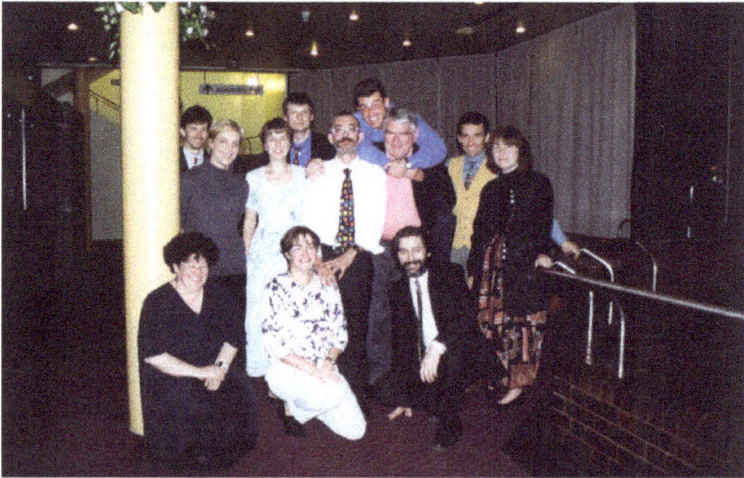

Reunion of trainees. From left to right: Bottom: Collette Coleman, Anne Godridge, Andrew Sykes, Carolyn Hall Middle: Christine Dumitresco, Isabel McCormick, Paco Fernandez, me, Simon Anderson. Back: Alan Kerry, Simon Acey, Norman Dawes.

Other trainees were: Mark Burgin, Mark Hammett, Bert van den Ende, Jutta Prekow, Patricio Coll, Mark Palmer, Adrian Rawlinson, Geeta Sahay, Sarah Bodey and Deborah Hewitt.

I do not have photographs of each of them and I apologise if I do not write something about everyone. They were all very competent doctors. I hope what I write about some of these fantastic doctors will capture the essence of the training relationship.

I had to wait six months until I would be allocated my first full-time trainee. Three months before that time, I received a phone call from Jeff, the course organiser, to tell me that one of the trainers (David Wilkinson) was not well and had to stop working. He asked me if I could take over David's trainee. I was very nervous about my first experience as a trainer. Isobel McCormick (see group photo above) came as my first trainee and, when we first talked together, said to me, "I am not sure I want to be a GP." That threw me.

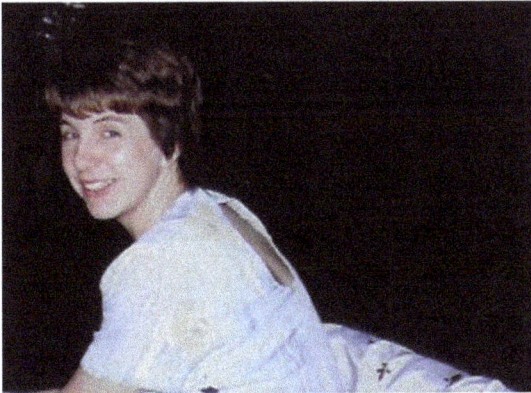

Isobel McCormick

At first the trainee was accompanied by the trainer on visits. Isobel was perfectly competent to go on visits on her own, having had three months' training in general practice already. I remember her returning from Fryston, the nearby pit village, looking somewhat fearful. She had met some of the Alsatians and other large dogs that wandered freely in the village.

Isobel's then husband worked for the Inland Revenue, and John Lee, my partner, got into the habit of whispering to me when we talked about the practice finances.

Isobel was a fantastic trainee and returned to us as a locum when Anne was on maternity leave. We are still in touch and she came for a coffee in 2018 to discuss her job situation. She has now retired, and I am sure she will have a fulfilled retirement.

In December 2018 Paco Fernandez stayed with me for a night, and I invited Bert and Hazel Bird (retired senior receptionist) for supper. I had not seen Paco for about twenty years and neither had I seen Bert for a long time. It was a lovely evening.

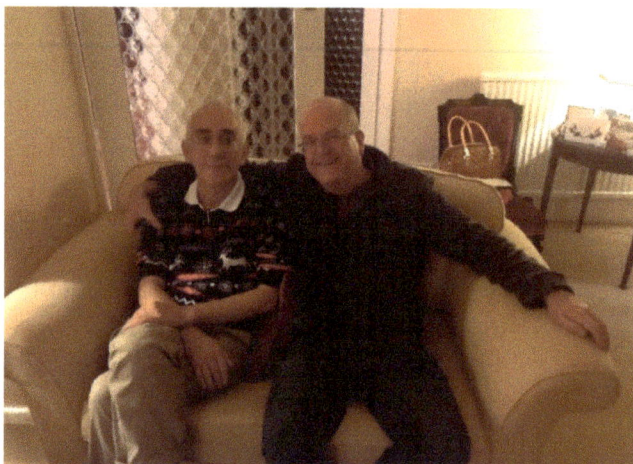

Paco and Bert 2018

Paco was and is a character. He gave up practicing medicine, became a Franciscan friar in Bolivia and has worked in China. He also worked on a beehive project for China while living in Hong Kong. He returned to Bolivia in 2019.

Paco was somewhat chaotic but is one of the kindest people I know. He was once arrested on the way to our surgery to do a locum. He was driving on the A1 dual carriageway and was running late. He decided to go onto the hard shoulder and put his foot down. A lorry driver reported him. The police stopped him, and there was a significant problem with his driving licence, so they took him to their police station.

Paco had some problems with the English language and sometimes I had difficulty making him understand certain things.

I once showed him an episode of Fawlty Towers where Basil Fawlty could not get his Spanish waiter, Manuel, to understand something. Basil said, "Let me explain," and then punched Manuel in the face! Paco found this amusing, thank goodness. I don't know what Jamie Bahrami would have thought of my doing that as a tutorial. On reflection, I do know. He would have laughed and pointed out the learning points on communication that could be discussed. I think most things have learning points.

Bert became an excellent GP. I undertook an interesting assessment of him. He became a partner in the practice in Pontefract where I was a patient. One time I consulted him there. He dealt with me in an exemplary manner. That was my final assessment. I was a bit cruel to him when he was about to move on from our practice. As a leaving present, I gave him a book on cockney rhyming slang. He had just become proficient in the English language. I think that was a rather poor joke.

I will digress. Tod Sloan was an American jockey born in 1874. He won many races in England and his name was lent to a cockney rhyming slang. He was always out front in his races – on his own. So the rhyming slang is: on your Tod. Tod Sloan; on your own. Get it? (Also, plates of meat – feet; Adam and Eve – believe ["I don't Adam and Eve you!"]. Have a look at http://www.cockneyrhymingslang.co.uk.)

Patricio Coll was another trainee who originated from Spain. He was in the Pontefract training scheme at the same time as Paco and they became friends. Patricio was a contrast to Paco. He was cool, calm and collected. One evening I was doing a shift for the out-of-hours GP service and Patricio came with me. We were on the shift doing visits. We had a request to visit a man who was in his room at a big hotel on the outskirts of Ossett. When we announced ourselves at reception, the receptionist started the process of registering us both for a room for the night.

Patricio later went back to Spain and got a job in one of the seaside holiday resorts, where his knowledge of the English language was a great asset.

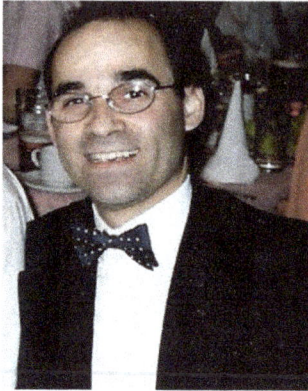

Patricio Coll

Christine Dumitrescu was trained in South Africa and is of Romanian background. It was a delight working with her. However, she was often late. I am always early. When I gave her a lift to a regional postgraduate committee meeting, we were even late for that. I mentioned this to Philip Nolan, one of the deputy directors of postgraduate GP education. He said it was a genetic problem. I have got the "early genes" and Christine the "late genes". He advised me not to mention it to her and think how I would feel if someone told me I had always to be late. I would have gone crazy.

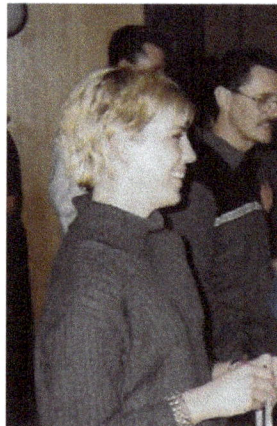

Christine Dumitrescu

Sarah Bodey is a Facebook friend of mine, so we can see what one another are up to. At the time Sarah was a trainee, the surgery premises became crowded. Sarah and I had to share a room, which was not ideal. She had recently had a baby and was breastfeeding. She used our room to express her breast milk. This is an example of the determination of women to become doctors in the sometimes non-understanding culture of male ambition.

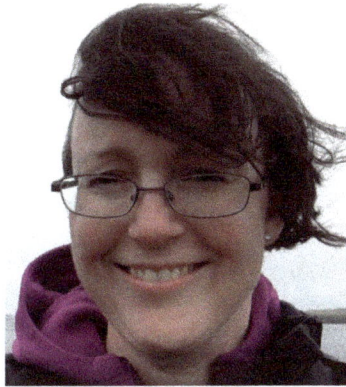

Sarah Bodey

Another ex-trainee who is a Facebook friend is Alan Kerry (see group photo).

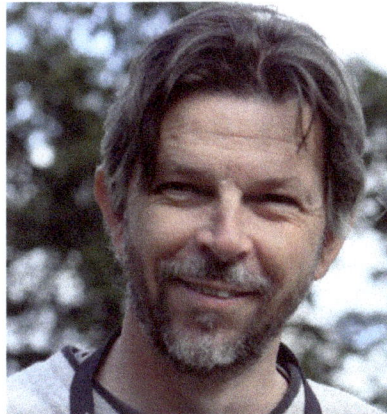

Alan Kerry

He lived in Ackworth, near Pontefract. Once, the practice went out to a pub for a murder mystery evening. One had to dress up. When Kath and I walked in, there was a glamorous woman with gorgeous legs sitting at the bar. It was Alan.

When he and Lisa moved to Leigh-on-Sea in Essex they called their house "Ackworth". After he had settled in as a GP there, they invited us to stay. I was impressed how much holiday Alan was allowed in his partnership agreement. I think it was eight weeks a year. Their firstborn had grown just tall enough to use a door handle, which she did for the first time while we were there. We had a trip to the coast and Alan took me on this horrifically frightening fairground big wheel thing. I vowed that I would pay him back for this experience and occasionally spend time looking up rides like that. Payback time might still happen. Alan has now retired.

Alan is one of the three doctors I have encountered here who, like me, were medical students at The London Hospital, Whitechapel. The first was the late Jean Wharton, a consultant gastroenterologist at Pontefract General Infirmary. The other is Linda Harris. She is the chief executive officer of a very successful company called Spectrum CIC, based in Wakefield. The company has a close link with a small charity, Spectrum People, which is based in the same building. I and Linda are fellow trustees of that charity, and it is good to meet her regularly. At one point, when Spectrum CIC was moving offices, it was based for a short time in Tieve Tara Medical Centre. Of course, we four from The London Hospital were the best of doctors.

Andrew Sykes (see group photo) was with us at the same time as Alan Kerry. They made good, good friends. Andrew and his wife, Gwennan, also lived in Ackworth. Gwennan did a locum for us, and we worked well together. She joined the Castleford Choral Society, of which my wife, Kath, and I were members. The society held a Patrons' evening once a year. Choir members entertained the patrons as way of saying thank you. One time, Gwennan and I performed a mouth organ duet. We entered the performance area with Gwennan carrying a huge cello case. Inside was her mouth organ.

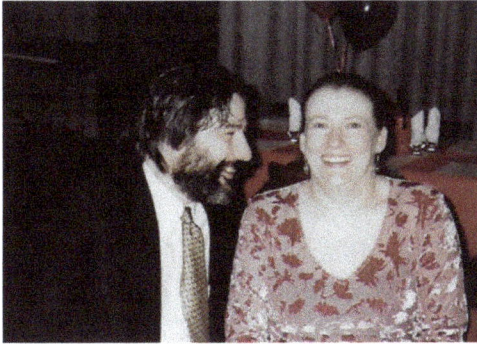

Andrew and Gwennan Sykes

Andrew became a GP in nearby Crofton and became chairman of the Wakefield and District Local Medical Committee. This is a committee which represents GPs and trainees. Carolyn Hall (see group photo) became the medical secretary of the LMC.

I once had a big argument with Andrew and John Lee, my partner. They were telling me what to wear at a dance. The invitation was for a "Black Tie" event. They said I should wear a black bow tie, and I said one could wear any colour of bow tie. I knew I was right! According to Debrett's Etiquette now, they were right. My apologies, boys. However, half the men wore coloured ties at that dance. They and I were the twinkle-toed dancing equivalents of the suffragettes.

Norman Dawes was great fun.

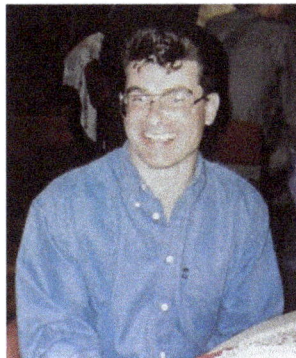

Norman Dawes

Andrea, one of the receptionists, used to knock on our consulting room doors and, when invited in, ask: "Any filin'?" I once knocked on Norman's door, and as I entered, he did a perfect imitation of Andrea, in a high-pitched voice, asking for files: "Any filin'?" At that time, we had an absolutely hopeless receptionist. At the end of a tutorial, Norman suggested we phone her and ask a question to see what her response would be so we could have a laugh. How cruel.

When my mother went into a nursing home, she let her bungalow to Norman. On Tuesday afternoons all trainees had to go to the postgraduate centre for the half-day training session. I decided one Tuesday afternoon, to pop up to my mother's bungalow, which should have been empty, and check all was OK. Norman was there relaxing watching the TV. He was playing truant.

Norman emigrated to New Zealand, and I occasionally see him when he is over here.

Mark Palmer became a GP in Rothwell, which is about six miles from Airedale. I have two memories of him that make me smile. The first was an occasion when we had to dress up and it was either at the murder mystery evening or another social event for the practice. Mark came as a cardinal and looked amazing. Instead of having a bible, he had the British National Formulary (BNF). This was the bible for doctors and contained detailed factual information about every drug one could prescribe. I kept one in my pocket when I was working as a houseman and in my doctor's bag when I was a GP.

My second memory of Mark took place in Florida. Kath and I often holidayed there and on one occasion drove down to the southern end of the peninsula – Key West, an area ninety miles from Cuba. We were at a viewing area for the amazing sunsets when we heard a voice shout out: "Richard!" It was Mark Palmer. We had no idea he would be there, and indeed I had not seen him for a number of years. We went out with him that evening for dinner.

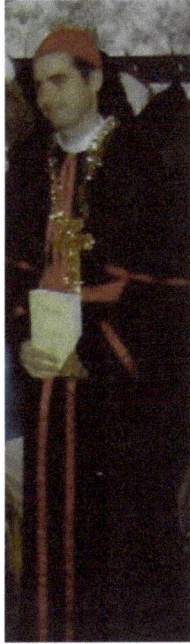

Cardinal Mark Palmer

Jutta Prekow is German. It was very interesting for me, as the son of a German mother, to be allocated a German trainee. Her CV stated her main hobby was the Argentine Tango. I missed the occasion at a practice party when she did a demonstration dance with her then partner, Sven. She got a job in Bradford and was so proud to pass the assessments to become a GP. To be excellent in consultation skills in a second language is amazing. I did try to headhunt her once without success.

She and Sven once invited me and Kath for a meal at their house. They gave tango dancing lessons in that medium sized house. The carpets could be rolled back and furniture moved so that there was a reasonable expanse of wooden flooring for practice. We communicate at Christmas and I really appreciated her coming to Kath's funeral.

Adrian Rawlinson was a very likeable person. He was positive about what he wanted to learn. He was an eligible bachelor, and some of the surgery staff took a shine to him. (That is a polite way of putting it. "Fancied" is a better word.) I found out after the event that one of the staff fixed him up a date with a patient. I am not sure of the ethics of that arrangement.

Towards the end of his attachment with us, Kath and I took him out for a meal and we ended up in the surgery's local pub, The Fryston Hotel, which was an eye-opener. I very rarely went into local pubs. My father advised me that a GP going into a pub where the patients lived could be very much frowned on by some, while others would think it was a great thing to do. Adrian once invited those working at the surgery to his flat in Leeds. I think we went for a meal out before that. I recollect that we were like a plague of locusts descending on the nibbles and drinks he provided us.

Adrian married an American and has lived and worked there for many years. He has a varied portfolio of skills and jobs. He is vice president of medical affairs at hims/hers – a company dealing with men's health problems and products. (Sounds like a dating agency to me.) He is a specialist in musculoskeletal medicine. We communicate with one another occasionally using LinkedIn.

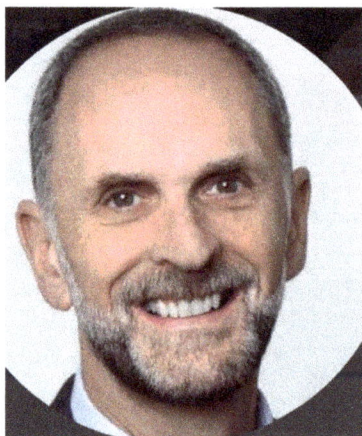

Adrian Rawlinson

Geeta Sahay became a partner of Ashgrove Surgery in Knottingley. Geeta is the wife of a local consultant gastroenterologist. I was so pleased when, at the end of her training with me, they came for a coffee and gave me a very generous present.

Mark Burgin was a very bright man who was educated at one of the Oxbridge colleges. He was one of the early trainees. He was rather eccentric and actually we did not click. Perhaps he was too bright – if that is possible. At the time of his stay with us, there was a push to wean patients off drugs such as Valium and Librium. After work, Mark altered the computer records of all such patients and labelled them as having a drug addiction problem. This came up on the first screen when the patient was brought up on the computer. We altered that.

Mark was with us over a winter. He was married to a midwife who worked locally. On one particularly snowy day, he phoned in before 9 am. He said he had thought hard about the ethics of his decision and had chosen to drive his wife to her home visits rather than come into work with us. I was furious. Perhaps he was right. Maybe I would have done the same.

Mark is a very successful doctor. He is a GP in Barnsley and an expert in medico-legal problems.

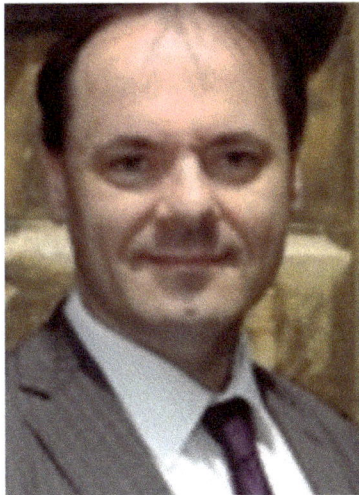

Mark Burgin

Round about the year 2000, I gave up training GPs in the practice but continued to be deeply involved with postgraduate GP education for a further ten years. I retired as a GP in 2005 after a couple of years dropping to three days a week. My first full-time six-month trainee attachment was with Anne Godridge, who is now the senior partner (see Chapter 4). I am so grateful to Anne Godridge for allowing me to develop my career in education. She could easily have objected and made me do more work in the practice. It was in February 2000 that Anne started as a trainer. I had the very strange experience of being the chair of the interviewing panel at the Yorkshire Deanery the time Anne was interviewed for her application. I remember having to tell Jamie Bahrami off during her interview. He was making too many jokes. He was the director of postgraduate GP education as I have already mentioned. She got through with flying colours. There were only four on the interviewing panel rather than the ten I had.

For many years it was expected that all practice personnel were involved in training. The trainee spent time with the health visitor, district nurse, practice manager and others. I did undertake some tutorials with Anne's trainees.

Despite being a most amiable person, Vijay Kumar drove me mad as he was often late for work. At one point I did not believe that the reason for his lateness was that the M62 was so busy. I nearly went to that motorway first thing one morning when I was on holiday to check it out. However, Vijay had a very sharp brain and became an excellent GP in Doncaster. He has had a stunning career and is provost of the Yorkshire Faculty of the Royal College of General Practitioners. (I was asked to take on that role many years ago but turned it down.) He is an honorary professor and a fellow of the Royal College of Surgeons. His wife is a GP in Knottingley.

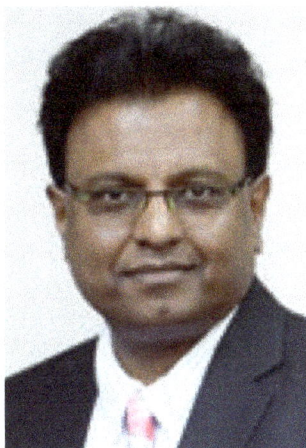

Vijay Kumar

Martin O'Hare was from Northern Ireland and was a very conscientious doctor. Anne had him as her trainee for two six-month periods, which was unusual. He became ill while working with us and had to retire. We lost touch with him. I really got on with him and hope he is well and happy.

Rosario Vega is Spanish and she eventually became a partner. She was a superb GP and we are Facebook friends. She left the practice a few years ago and became a partner in Pontefract (see Chapter 4).

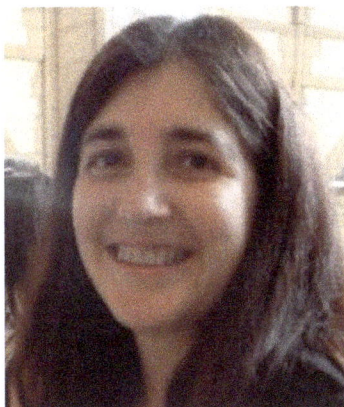

Rosario Vega

Sean Allen and Soumitra Dutta became partners in Wakefield District practices. Ben Young was trained by Anne and was a very popular GP partner of Tieve Tara. There were a lot of patients who were upset when he left in 2018 to join a practice nearer where he lived. Samra Abbas and Maryam Almassi were also a delight to work with.

I had twenty-two trainees and Anne has trained thirty-two so far (January 2019). That is a huge number of doctors who have been trained in Tieve Tara Surgery/Medical Centre. At one point about four or so years ago, each partner in the practice had been trained there. Airedale is a very difficult area in which to work as a GP. I am convinced that it is the culture of the practice that results in a significant number of trainees wanting to stay.

I had two other training experiences at Tieve Tara.

Sarah Baker had been working a in a senior NHS management job in Leeds for a number of years, as I mentioned in Chapter 4. I was asked to take her on for familiarisation training. She very quickly came up to the mark. She became a partner for a short while.

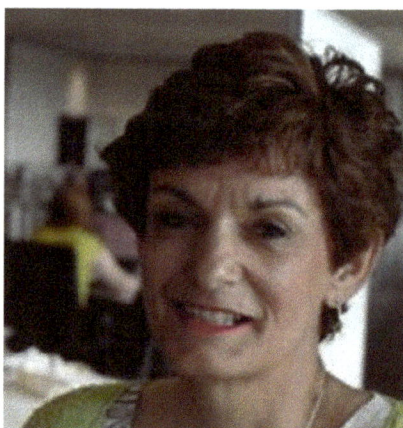

Sarah Baker

Jackie Spencer, also previously mentioned, was our district nurse and applied to Huddersfield University to undertake a masters' degree to become a nurse practitioner. I became her practice tutor. The two years' training was comprehensive, and she had to learn how to examine patients just like we doctors. I had what might be a unique experience for a male doctor. She asked me to be her chaperone while she examined a man's testicles. I actually felt awkward. I don't think health professionals think much about how chaperones feel.

We occasionally had to go together for afternoons of training. I realised that those were the only occasions I had actually been out with a nurse. This is a rare thing for male medical students/doctors. Many of my male medical friends married nurses.

Jackie had excellent consultation skills and wrote a very good dissertation. After she qualified, she became a nurse practitioner in a general practice in Knottingley. She specialised in mental health there.

This book is not about my career, and so I will just write that one of the loves of my professional career was teaching. I became a Continuing Medical Education GP tutor for Pontefract. I was also the course organiser for GP trainees there but only for a short time. At one time these two jobs overlapped with each other and with my being a trainer. I eventually became an associate director of postgraduate GP education. I worked closely with Jamie Bahrami, the director, at the Yorkshire Deanery based in Leeds University. This was a privilege. He is one of my medical heroes. I worked briefly with his successor, George Taylor, and ended my postgraduate education career as education advisor to the district's Primary Care Trust. I continued in that role for five years.

At my interview for Associate Director, I said that it was a privilege to be a doctor. To be a doctor and a teacher as well was an even greater privilege. I was so lucky.

Chapter 7 – Patients

This is a difficult chapter to write for several reasons. There is the ethical problem of confidentiality that all doctors should respect, even after a patient's death.

I don't want anecdotes and amusing experiences to dominate the chapter. However, the experiences of most doctors include very funny situations. These situations might not be at all amusing to the patient, however.

I really appreciate having dealt with the same patients in Airedale for twenty-seven years. This is called continuity of care, which is generally accepted, other things being equal, to have a positive effect on health and life expectancy. Continuity of care is disappearing because of the new ways of helping patients and the pressure of work on GPs and the NHS in general. Both patients and GPs regret this situation.

Many of my friends from childhood joined the practice, as did friends and patients of my parents. This was a fantastic thing for them to do. However, looking after friends as a doctor has disadvantages for both as I will describe later.

I have appreciated the strength of the doctor–patient relationship since I retired from general practice in 2005. There is a friendship aspect of the relationship that can be there for life. I love meeting ex-patients when I am out and about. They usually sum up their health problems but no longer ask my opinion on these. We talk about families, memories and life in general. I like going for a walk in the local pit village of Fryston. Recently there was a youngish man at his front door, and I was some distance away. He shouted out, "Oi. Sloany." I went up to him and we had a chat and a laugh together. Some men I meet call me "love", which is a common thing to do in the north.

When I was a child, in the school holidays I often accompanied my mother or father on their visits. I stayed in the car. There were not great distances to drive and often three or more home visits could be made with the car parked in the same spot. Sometimes, there were terribly foggy days, and on one such day, in the evening, my father walked a mile to a visit request. When my father arrived, he was told it would have been OK if he had come the next day. When he got to his early sixties, he had a unique method of driving in the fog. He drove very slowly on the wrong side of the road because he could see the kerb more easily.

Just before Christmas my mother would go out and take mince pies and small presents for the patients she knew who were very poor. I once went with her. She pulled up at a house in Fryston. It was dark and there were no lights on in the house. When my mother returned to her car, she explained that the couple who lived there were both blind. This couple joined my practice very early on and were a pleasure for me to help. Their daughter is a Facebook friend.

Uncle Sam (my father's brother) was a GP in Wakefield, and I stayed with him and Aunty Agnes once a week. It was on the day I attended scouts at Wakefield Grammar School, where I was a pupil. I sometimes was with them in the daytime and would go out with Uncle Sam on his visits. He had made himself a fascinating gadget. It was a pair of gloves with a heating filament embedded in the material. He could plug these gloves into the car's cigar lighter and they warmed up like a mini electric blanket. His hands were never cold when he examined a patient. He also wore a beret for the visits, which I never quite understood. He was a very smartly dressed man. I really loved him and my aunt such a lot. I used to say to my parents, "I like Wakefield better than England." Geography was never a strength of mine.

My parents had what some called "front door patients". They never came to the surgery but were seen in the house. Some of these patients were their friends. Some of the children of these families became my friends and some became my patients after 1978. However, in contrast to my parents, I did not see patients in the private house. This had the effect that one of those friends of my parents never came to the surgery in more than twenty years! Actually, there was one friend I did see in my house. Grahame and

I were fellow medical students and we met at University College London in 1963. He became a GP in Pontefract, which is about 4 miles from me. He was my GP and I his. We are close friends to this day. We saw one another about our medical problems in our homes.

Does a GP establish relationships with patients that result in true friendships? I certainly became close friends with the Bullingham family when I was a GP in Cheltenham. Bill Bullingham was a patient. However, I think the friendship developed from an introduction made at a social occasion by my GP partner, Robin Harrod. I am godfather to Rachael, Bill and Anna Bullingham's daughter. (I am also godfather to Samantha, Robin and Christine's daughter.)

**

Kath and I had a special relationship with two patients whom I did not know before I returned to Castleford in 1978. These relationships evolved into friendships. Instead of using taxis when we were going out to friends or restaurants etc., we asked a patient to drive us in his car. I think this was something I picked up from Bill Bullingham in Cheltenham.

The first, who I know would wish to remain anonymous, had a significant illness which resulted from his time in the armed forces. He was totally reliable and drove us for years. After an evening out, we invited him into our house and we sat and chatted for up to an hour. I drove a four-wheel drive Fiat Panda for years, and in the end he used to service it for me. One evening, I broke down on the A1 dual carriageway and was in what looked, at first sight, like the middle of nowhere. I noticed that across the road was a sign for a footpath to the village of Micklefield. I did not have a mobile phone and neither did I have any money. It was becoming dark. After about twenty minutes, I arrived in Micklefield and went into the pub and explained the situation to the landlord. He let me use the phone and gave me half a pint of beer. I phoned our driver and he came out and recued me. We had that car for ten years and when we decided to buy another, we gave it to the driver as a present. I have since lost touch with him. I last saw him at his home about three years ago.

The second patient was Kevin Tansley (nicknamed Liver). He again was also so reliable. The only time he could not take us was when there was a home rugby game for Castleford. He was a retired miner and was active in the miners' strike of 1984/5. He got arrested on one occasion. I could book him using texts. Early one morning, he was uncharacteristically late, and I was in a bit of a panic as I had to catch a train. He turned up and was wearing his pyjamas. He had slept in.

The occasion we reminisced about many times was one where he had taken Kath and me to Pontefract for dinner at our friends' house. I definitely had too much to drink that evening. Kevin dropped us off at our house and drove off. I had come home in George Gauden's jacket. I had no house keys and neither did I have my electronic diary with Kevin's phone number. Kath was absolutely livid, and I don't blame her. Fortunately, one of the hosts, Sue Smith, got my phone and remembered Kevin's name. He went to Pontefract and got my jacket and then came back to our house. After that, on many occasions when we were coming home from somewhere, he would enquire if I had the right jacket.

Kevin was one of the kindest men I have known. He regularly took an elderly friend of Kath's, Molly Healey, to the vet with her virtually blind dog. Once, a friend of mine, Liz Wheeldon, phoned me on my mobile in the evening when I was staying at Heathrow Airport before a holiday. She was not well and wanted to get her son home from hospital in Leeds. Kevin dropped everything and took Liz to Leeds and sorted things out for her.

Kevin developed an oesophageal cancer. I know that all who knew him were devastated at this news. I was in touch with his wife, Kathryn, both by text and on Facebook. I visited two or three times during his final illness. I said something to him on a visit very shortly before he died, and he smiled. He died just before Christmas 2019.

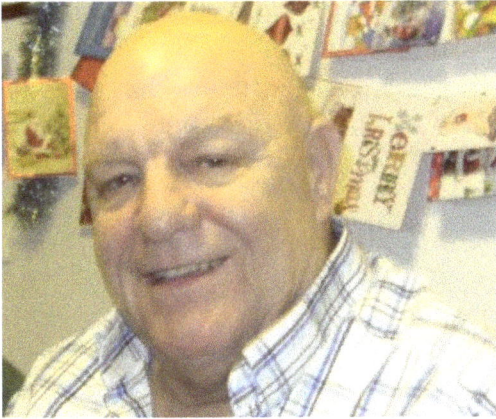

Kevin Tansley

* * *

As I mentioned earlier, in 1978, when my wife, Kath, and I started up the practice from scratch, a significant number of my old friends and people I knew in my youth joined our practice. I always worried when consulting with a friend. Did I over-investigate? Was my consultation style different? Did I spend more time with them than the others? I certainly did worry more about my friends who were patients than the patients who were not my friends. I worried about the latter as well. That made me feel guilty. It was strongly recommended that GPs should treat everyone in the same way. It had been shown in one study that GPs spent more time in consultations with educated middle-class patients than with working-class patients. That is not regarded as good practice. I found it very difficult to apply that standard to my friends. I certainly treated each patient with the same respect and professionalism irrespective of education, class, race, etc.

I rarely gave out my private telephone number to a patient. Of course, my friends had my private number, and some were my patients. I told my oldest friend, George, that he could phone me any time. On one occasion, my wife, Kath, and I were staying with friends in Cheltenham and I went off to refuel my car. My mobile phone rang while I was at the pump, and it was George. He had a very painful infected throat. I said to him, "Do you know where I am? I am at a garage in Cheltenham." George replied: "You can phone a chemist, can't you?" Actually, I think he was somewhat politer than that. I did phone a chemist and prescribed antibiotics. (The routine prescribing of antibiotics for sore throats is out of fashion now.)

When I was on holiday in Italy about ten years after I retired, I had a call on my mobile phone. It was a man asking for an appointment at the surgery! I explained where I was and that I was retired. He was not at all pleased. I must have given him my telephone number when I was looking after one of his family. I did give my private phone number to the families of patients who were dying at home. He had probably kept it on his phone for all those years. He rang again for another appointment a couple of days later!

* * *

The amusing situations all doctors come across keep us sane. We are not smiling or laughing at misfortune. Finding the funny side of things is a psychological release method for doctors and nurses dealing with the most awful problems. There was always a lot of laughter in A & E departments.

In the early days, we ran open surgeries and patients would queue up in the reception area. There was a man who often tried to jump the queue by "collapsing" to the floor. I fell for this at first, but he gave it up when I used to just step over him and call the next patient.

Martin Raftery (nicknamed Stursh – we called him Raftery) was a retired coal miner and veteran of the Second World War. He and his wife, Maud, were our next-door neighbours and were also patients. They became friends of ours. Their house was a council house with a large, well-kept garden. Have a look at the 1981 aerial photo of the house and surgery in Chapter 1. The Rafterys' house is clearly seen on the left of the photo. Maud lived there when she was a child. Her mother, Mrs. Bruin, kept geese and I used to watch them through a gap in the fence.

Raftery made himself a gate through the fence separating our gardens. He looked after our dogs and the house when we were away. He and Maud owned a cat. One day when he was out for a walk, Raftery came across the cat, which had been run over. He was really upset. He took the cat home and buried it in the garden. Later, when he was having a cup of tea and crying, a cat walked into the room. It was his cat! He exclaimed with delight, "I've just buried thee!" He had buried someone else's cat.

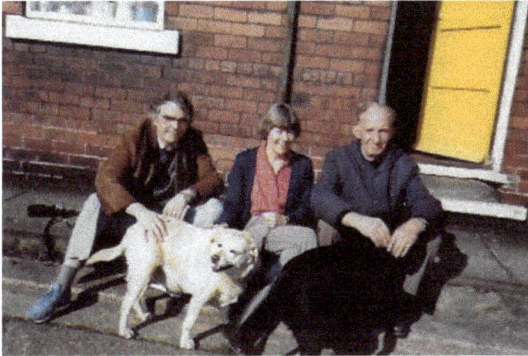

Me, Kath, Raftery, Sindy (golden) and Sam

We had a pond with goldfish and one of them died. We were leaving for a holiday. We said goodbye to Raftery, who had come to look after the dogs. I looked in the rear-view mirror of the car and saw Raftery with the dead goldfish in the palm of his hand. He was blowing at its head to try and revive it. He was a very kind man.

Raftery fell out with me for not removing a splinter from his finger when he asked me. He never spoke to me, Kath or Maureen, our housekeeper, for the rest of his life. He nailed up the gate between our gardens. I should have apologised. I really should. However, I found out he stopped speaking to one of his close friends years ago. He had been in the army with him in the Second World War.

Maud was an ex-policewoman and she was also very kind to us. Soon after we arrived at Tieve Tara house we bought a second-hand cooker. Kath was cooking the first Sunday roast of our marriage. Suddenly the cooker failed and Kath was in tears. The doorbell rang and there was Maud and another neighbour, Waveney Brain. It was a coincidence that they just arrived then. They fixed it in a minute or two.

I think it is a very rare thing for a GP to live next door to a council house and make friends like that. All of our neighbours became patients. They were and still are fantastic neighbours who I regard as friends, some as good friends.

* * *

I once did a repeat home visit to an elderly man and we had a fairly long conversation as to how his legs were feeling. He said they were coming on nicely. I realised after a while I did not know him from Adam. I had gone into the house next door by mistake. This happened again a few years later with another patient. I rang the doorbell, and the man was upstairs on the lavatory. He shouted for me to sit down and that he would not be long. When he came downstairs, I realised my error. My patient was next door. Most GPs I know have had these experiences.

I was particularly grumpy one afternoon. I was on call and a man phoned the surgery requesting a home visit. I said to him, "Do you realise that in the USA and Germany there is no such thing as a home visit?" He replied "Well! This is bloody England!" I went. Urgent home visit requests just before a surgery are really disrupting and stressful.

* * *

Jack Hulme was a famous Yorkshire photographer and he lived in Fryston, the pit village less than half a mile from the surgery and house. His books of photographs of life in Fryston village were published. He took photographs of me and my parents when I was a child. He took photos at my birthday parties. There is one photograph taken by him in Chapter 1. He was invited to be the official photographer at the opening ceremony for an early extension of the surgery.

Jack had a fireguard in front of his television table. This puzzled me. He explained that when there was a football match, the dog repeatedly lunged towards the screen to try and get the ball.

After Jack died a blue plaque was affixed to his house. His grandson, Trevor Moorby, has thousands of his grandfather's photos and sent me some of me and my parents from when I was a child. Trevor is a Facebook friend.

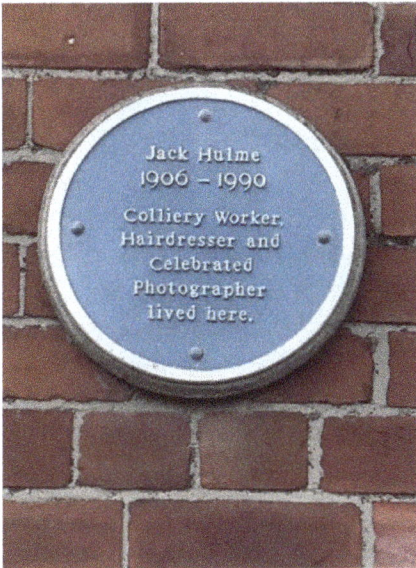

The blue plaque

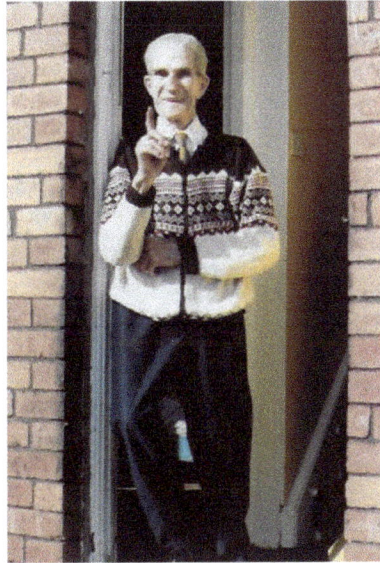

Jack Hulme

* * *

We called patients to our consulting rooms using the phone connected to a loudspeaker in the waiting room. Once, I called "Mrs. Smith to room 2, please. Mrs. Smith to room 2." There was a brief knock on the door, the patient entered and the first thing said was, "Actually, I'm a crow." She had married and her name was now Crow.

One day, I saw a patient in the morning, and on his way out, he booked another appoinment for the afternoon because he had forgotten to tell me something. No wonder it is difficult to get an appointment.

I was once asked to visit to a woman who had a chest infection. Three minutes after I had left the house, I had a call on my mobile phone. It was her husband wanting me to visit again because he had "started with it".

Over the years, we encountered what we called "heartsink patients". Some of these patients are demanding, some irritating and some are playing a complex psychological game. One patient would say "I don't know. I really don't know," or something similar, to almost every question I asked her.

"How are you, Mrs. Jones?"

"Well, I don't really know, doctor. I really don't know. "

"Did the new tablets help with your indigesion?"

"I don't know, doctor. I really don't know."

She developed a terminal disease shortly before I retired. She was one of two patients I continued visiting after I retired. I am not sure why I did that. I could not prescribe or practice medicine anymore. What was fascinating was that my relationship with her changed. There were no time restraints, and I settled into a comfy chair and had long pleasant conversations with her and her husband, who was also ill. The feeling of my heart sinking disappeared. I attended her funeral.

There was a male patient who was a very good singer. He died. A relation came to see me and I asked how things were. She said, "Did you know he sang at his own funeral?" It was a recording, of course.

A man who had had his arm amputated below the shoulder could tie his shoelaces up with his remaining hand. If we had time, I used to ask him to show me as it was fascinating. I have no idea how he did that. I should have videoed it. There was no such thing as YouTube then. Have a look at this: https://youtu.be/CLqdQ-f1RO0.

There was a patient who maintained that his parrot could forecast the weather. It obviously learned this from the television. However, he and the parrot were on the local news on one occasion and the parrot seemed to not just be repeating random forecasts but actually getting it right! However, one can't be wrong too many times if one says it will rain.

Pigeon fancying and racing were significant hobbies in Airedale. Pigeon fancying is breeding and keeping pigeons. This has been going on for 10,000 years. There were pigeon huts not so far from Tieve Tara, and some of these pigeons had their own guard dog. One pigeon owner had read that a certain cough medicine perked them up and asked if I would give him a prescription for some. I did not.

Late one night I went out into our garden and spotted an owl on the garage roof. Then I heard a loud whisper: "Come here. Oi, come here." A neighbour had a pet owl that he only let out late at night.

Another patient had about sixty budgerigars. He developed a chronic cough. I thought it was to do with the birds. I referred him to a consultant, but it turned out not to be related to his pets.

* * *

When I was a child, there were several sweet and liquorice factories in Castleford and Pontefract. Some sweets were deformed by the manufacturing process. Sometimes employees were given the defects to take home. Occasionally, a bag of these sweets was given to my parents and ended up with me. (No wonder I was overweight as a youth.) Some of these factories were still active when I started work at Tieve Tara Surgery in 1978. There are liquorice factories in Pontefract now. In the early 1980s, I had a woman see me who had dropped a very heavy bag of liquorice torpedoes onto her foot, which caused a significant injury. I advised her to take a couple of weeks off work, and it amused me to write on her medical certificate the reason she could not work: "Injury to right foot from falling heavy container of liquorice torpedoes". GPs felt that no one ever read what was written on these certificates. I saw in a medical journal that a GP had certified a patient not fit for work on repeated occasions. The reason he stated for the illness was "Plumbum pendulum". That is Latin for lead-swinging!

One patient tried to persuade me to join the Jehovah's Witnesses and brought the magazine "Awake" to each consultation. He did this for a number of years. In the end I said to him that if he was able to prove 100 per cent that the Jehovah's Witnesses was the only true religion, I still would not join. When he asked why not, I said, "Narrow-minded." He continued to see me regularly and never mentioned Jehovah's Witnesses or brought the Awake magazine again. He was a very kind person and we did not fall out.

* * *

Of course it was really upsetting for me when a patient died, and I sometimes went to the funeral. I might have known the patient for decades. I had great difficulty when, in the middle of a consultation, I had popped down to reception to get something and was told of the death of a patient. I had to reign back my emotions and go back to my consulting room and continue as though nothing had happened. I answered my phone in the middle of a consultation because I was worried about one of our best friends, who was very ill. His son, James, had called to tell me his father, our friend, had died. I carried on with the consultation as though nothing had happened. I broke down in the evening at a trainers' meeting. I did my evening surgery as usual the day my mother had died in the afternoon (an expected death).

Terminal care was particularly rewarding. Making a patient comfortable and pain-free with drugs, a compassionate approach and the help of one's partners, the district and Macmillan nurses was a privilege. This was true family doctoring. It was sometimes mentally exhausting. One Christmas time I had three cases on the go, including one man I knew particularly well. My partners agreed that we should never do this level of terminal care again. That care included going to see the patient when one was off duty and sometimes giving out one's private phone number.

* * *

My mother was a patient of the practice and was a diabetic on insulin. (I too am a diabetic. I blame my diabetes on my mother. Actually, I blame everything on my mother!) She never came to our diabetic clinic but dealt with her diabetes over the phone with her close colleague, John Turner, a consultant physician (see chapter on associates). When I asked her why she did not come to the clinic, she replied: "I like to be dealt with by people who know what they are talking about."

* * *

Where there has been continuity of care in a practice, a GP can get to know his patients and their families very well over several decades. Towards the end of my general practice career, I dealt with more and more psychiatric problems. Patients I had got to know over the years did not want to start from scratch with another doctor. I enjoyed that work very much.

Sometimes patients were very disturbed indeed and threatening violence. If called to a situation that could be dangerous I parked my car outside, left the door open and the igntion key in place. We once had a psychopath who broke the treatment room window by headbutting it. I saw him later in the police station. I was nervous and asked if someone could accompany me and remain in the cell while I did the assessment. A policewoman was called. I thought it should have been a man. I was mistaken; male patients seem to calm down when confronted by women officers. On another occasion, a patient was running amock in the surgery. We called the police and a policewoman came and sorted things out.

* * *

Castleford was a coal mining town and it would be remiss of me not to write about the special qualities and medical problems of the miners and ex-miners.

When my mother heard I was returning to Airedale as a GP she advised me that the two things I ought to be familiar with in detail were chest diseases and athlete's foot. Pneumoconiosis (dust disease), bronchitis and emphysema were common in coal miners, who often smoked cigarettes as well as being exposed to awful and dusty conditions down the mines. Athlete's foot was common because the miners always showered at the pit after a shift. After the miners' strike ended in 1985, Fryston Pit was closed down. Of course the miners were not only sad but also very angry. When my mother heard the pit was closing she said, "Thank goodness. It was the most unhealthy place imaginable." She was the only person I have come across who was pleased by the pit closures.

There was the most amazing community spirit during that strike. People helped one another out, much as they are doing now in the coronavirus pandemic of 2020. The women were used to looking afer their children when they had minor illnesses and fevers. The men were not and panicked somewhat when their children became ill. The fathers insisted their children were seen by a doctor. There was significantly more anxiety and depression as well as new poverty. Patients could not afford to go to the dentist, and one man lost 2 stones in weight because his teeth were so painful that he could not eat properly. These families will never forgive or forget that strike and its effect on this community.

* * *

I retired as a GP in 2005 and still (as of 2020) live in the house next to the surgery (Hill House). I am a Facebook addict. I have a significant number of ex-patients as Facebook friends and a similarly significant number wanting to become a friend. It actually has got a bit out of hand. I have always been an IT nut (but not quite a nerd). I think Facebook, Twitter, WhatsApp, etc. are great ways to communicate, if used properly.

Of course, I am a patient too. Since my friend Grahame (my GP) retired at about the same time as me, I have no particular perks in the NHS. Indeed, Kath and I changed to a Castleford practice where I knew most of the GPs well. Like everyone, I have trouble getting an appointment with the GP of my choice. Continuity of care is therefore being eroded. This is not so in the private sector as regards seeing a consultant. It was not good for one to be a patient at the practice where one worked. However, in March 2019 I changed doctor and returned to Tieve Tara Medical Centre. This was mainly because I was on the Patient Participation Panel as an advisor and wanted to be a proper member as a patient. I have had excellent management from my old practice.

I do not miss working as a GP at all. I am so lucky to be involved with voluntary groups and a couple of charities all trying to help the most vulnerable people in the Wakefield district.

2003 was the twenty-fifth anniversary of my being a GP at Tieve Tara Surgery. There was a dedicated and hard-working Patient Participation Group then. To my utter surprise, they produced a celebratory booklet entitled "Born to be a Doctor" and also arranged a party. I have not got many photographs of patients and I particularly like this one from the book.

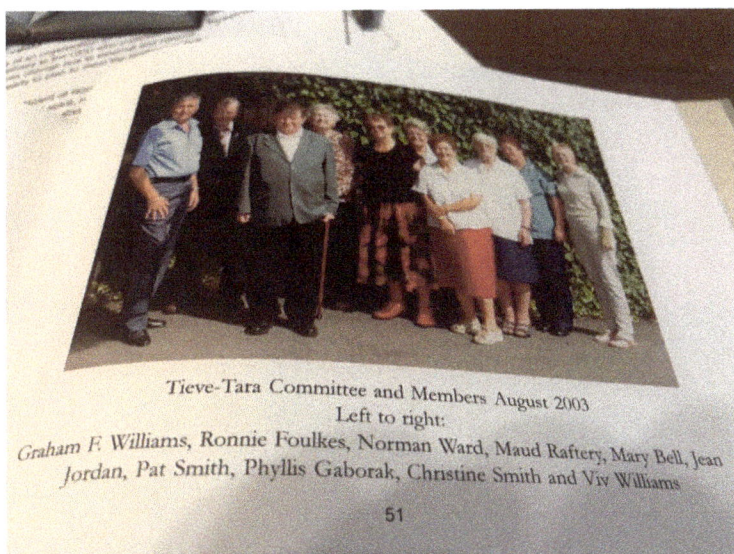

Tieve-Tara Committee and Members August 2003
Left to right:
Graham F. Williams, Ronnie Foulkes, Norman Ward, Maud Raftery, Mary Bell, Jean Jordan, Pat Smith, Phyllis Gaborak, Christine Smith and Viv Williams

51

The Patients' Participation Group 2003

I, my late wife and parents owe such a lot to the patients and people of Airedale and Castleford.

Afterword

The afterword is a final piece written by the author often showing developments after a book is completed.

I thought I had completed this book in the summer of 2019. However, I discovered that the medical practice was in trouble. I am a member of the Patient Participation Group, and we had meetings with the practice. The problems were described to us in general terms.

I also met one of the partners, Deborah Hewitt, in my house and she explained things in more detail. As I wrote earlier in this book, I have always highly respected her opinion. She decided to resign but came back as a locum one day a week.

We were told that a rescue operation would be led by Dr. Linda Harris FRCGP, Chief Executive of Spectrum CIC (Community Interest Company). I was delighted at this move. I have known Linda for many years. Indeed, we are fellow trustees of the charitable arm of her company, Spectrum People.

Partners resigned and the nurse practitioner became sick. Eventually, that left one partner, Anne Godridge, holding the fort along with very expensive locums. I think they charge about £800 a day or more. The practice had also drifted into having financial problems. We all know Anne has been a star. Mind you, she had a decent trainer!

At the time of writing this (May 2020), the information I have is that Spectrum CIC is considering having a formal agreement to jointly manage the practice, and the practice is advertising for a partner.

The crisis in the practice combined with the Covid-19 pandemic has resulted in the medical centre adopting completely different and modern working practices. This has happened in all general practices throughout the UK.

This is how I see the future of the practice after Anne has retired (which I think will be in the not too distant future):

The practice website is superb with lots of information and facilities to order repeat prescriptions and make appointments. There is a facility where documents can be uploaded and a question asked or a problem described. Then, in the fullness of time, the appropriate person will get back to the patient. This facility will be developed further, I am sure. There will be more teleconsultations (phone and video) and the option to communicate by email.

The Patient Participation Group will have members that truly represent the diversity of the patients and will communicate by email, in person and by teleconferencing.

The practice will have a comprehensive relationship with the local and district voluntary sector as well as elected local councillors. This will enable full engagement with appropriate social prescribing. Some of this social prescribing will be at no cost to the practice or neighbouring practices.

There will be a thriving relationship with other general practices looking after patients in Airedale, and patients will be able to consult with specialists (including GPs with special skills) in any of the Airedale Medical Centres or in practices further afield.

Medication will be delivered to some people using drones.

The practice will be a hub for the training of primary care workers for the area using the rooms at the end of the extension in the education suite. It is fortunate that the practice has a large car parking area.

Voice recognition will be sophisticated and will be used to update or make summaries of patient records. These records will be available on tablets and will be able to be accessed by healthcare workers anywhere. There should be significant working from home.

There will be a small laboratory to undertake the measurement of samples taken for simple investigations – blood tests, urine samples, etc. This facility has existed in Germany for over forty years. There will be in-house X-ray facilities in Airedale.

There will be a minivan to help patients access the medical centre and neighbouring practices.

There will be regular sessions for groups of patients for familiarisation with the internet. Tablets (iPads) will be loaned to patients or their relations to help with home consultations with acutely ill patients.

Staff and patients will be involved in a local TV channel which will transmit health prevention and other medical information to the people of Castleford. There will be live question time programmes on this channel. There will also be a dedicated local radio station with music for the younger population interspersed with health education material.

This medical practice has survived since the early 1920s. It has survived through many re-organisations of general practice.

Anne, with the help of Linda and others, has ensured that this general practice will survive for many more decades.

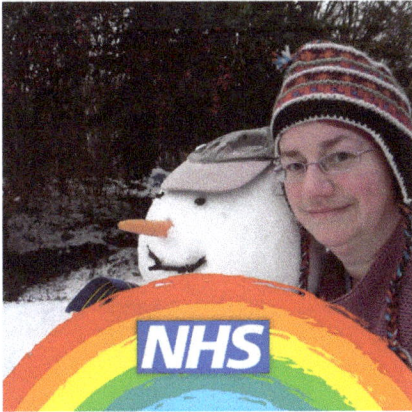

Anne Godridge 2020

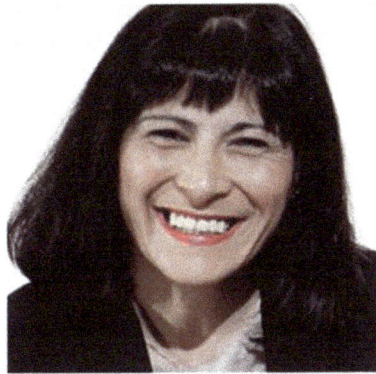

Linda Harris

Index

www.ingramcontent.com/pod-product-compliance
Lightning Source LLC
Chambersburg PA
CBHW040418110426
42813CB00013B/2698